Fundamental Aspects of
Tissue Viability Nursing

Bridget Günnewicht and Cheryl Dunford

Quay Books
MA Healthcare Limited

Quay Books Division, MA Healthcare Limited, Jesses Farm, Snow Hill, Dinton, Salisbury, Wiltshire, SP3 5HN

British Library Cataloguing-in-Publication Data
A catalogue record is available for this book

© MA Healthcare Limited 2004
ISBN 1 85642 260 7

Printed in Cromwell Press, Trowbridge

Contents

Chapter 4 Specific wound types 42

Foreword

Tissue viability has only been recognised as a specialist area of care for about twenty-five years, partially with the founding of the Tissue Viability Society in the United Kingdom (UK). Since then, nurses have been the main drivers for developing the specialty and there are currently about 500 specialist nurses in the UK. Many universities run specialist courses at Diploma and Bachelor level and there are even some at Masters level, thus adding legitimacy to the specialty. For those of us involved in tissue viability, these have been exciting times.

However, tissue viability is also a fundamental aspect of nursing care. At some point during their career, all nurses will care for patients with wounds or at risk of pressure ulcer development. Although not all nurses will seek to gain specialist knowledge of the topic, all nurses should have a fundamental understanding of how to care for these patients and how to utilise strategies for preventing pressure ulcers. The authors of this book have applied their considerable practical experience and knowledge to providing a useful text aimed at the novice nurse and those who wish to gain greater understanding of the fundamentals of tissue viability.

Although developments in tissue viability have been predominantly led by nurses, it still needs a multidisciplinary approach. I believe that readers will find this reflected within this book, along with a wide range of information on wounds of all types. The reflective activities and patient scenarios provide opportunities for the reader to reflect on what has been learnt.

I am pleased to recommend this book.

Carol Dealey
Birmingham
April, 2004

Introduction

This book provides a sound foundation in the field of tissue viability, particularly for those who are becoming involved in this aspect of nursing for the first time as a student or newly qualified nurse. The term tissue viability practitioner is used throughout this book to describe any nurse involved in providing care relating to tissue viability.

The care of patients with wounds is a rewarding area of nursing, but it can also be bewildering with the ever-expanding range of products and technologies available. A clear understanding of the fundamental aspects of tissue viability will prove invaluable.

Nurses are key stakeholders in the field of tissue viability, both in the delivery of care and advancement of the speciality, and need to take this responsibility seriously. The amount of money spent in 1999 in the United Kingdom (UK) on modern wound care products alone was £80,000,000 (Russell, 2002). Indeed, most of the new developments in technologies and dressings are considerably more expensive than traditional products. Nurses working in this field need to be able to justify the application of these through sound reasoning and measurement of outcomes.

Despite the advent of clinical guidelines and benchmarks there still remains a need for a stronger evidence base for much of this subject. Collaborative working between the many interested parties in tissue viability from patients, clinicians and manufacturers can help drive forward developments and initiatives to a greater extent.

We should always aim to provide the optimum environment for the patient to heal. This theme is central to the book. Throughout each chapter are patient scenarios, reflective activities and time-out sections. These are intended to allow you to focus directly on the patient who is central to all that we do. There will always be a number of patients for whom total wound healing and rehabilitation are not achievable outcomes. Although quality of life issues are important for all patients, they are vital for this group.

A core question is: what information do I need to nurse this patient? This information will include current evidence available on diagnosis, assessment and management approaches. Cue questions, such as those below, will help focus on the patient experience (Johns and Burford, 2000).

⌘ What meaning does this health event have for this person?
⌘ How is this person feeling?
⌘ How has this event affected their usual lifestyle and roles?
⌘ What support does this person have in life?
⌘ How does this person view the future for themselves and others?
⌘ What can I do to help this person?

This book will foster in the reader a strong interest in tissue viability. It is an exciting, challenging and rewarding aspect of health care and worthy of your attention.

Cheryl Dunford
Bridget Günnewicht
April, 2004

References

Johns C, Burford NDU (2000) Model reflective cues. In: *Becoming a Reflective Practitioner*. Blackwell Science, Oxford

Russell L (2002) Understanding physiology of wound healing and how dressings help. In: White RJ, ed. *Trends in Wound Care, volume I*. Quay Books, MA Healthcare Limited, Dinton, Salisbury

Chapter 1

How wounds heal

Overview of the healing process

Wound healing is a complex dynamic process about which there is still much to be discovered. To understand some of the fundamentals as to how wounds heal, the tissue viability practitioner needs a basic knowledge of the integumentary system which is composed of the skin and the structures that lie within it. The skin has two outer layers, the epidermis and dermis over a deeper layer known variously as the hypodermis, the superficial fascia or subcutaneous layer. This deeper layer is firmly attached to the outer skin layers, but is also anchored securely to underlying tissues and organs (Brooker, 1993).

The epidermis

This is the superficial, thinner outer layer, composed of epithelial tissue and is itself subdivided into five layers. The epidermis does not have a blood supply (it is avascular).

The dermis

This layer is deeper, thicker and is composed of connective tissue. It contains collagen, elastic fibres and blood vessels. The junction between the dermis and epidermis is an area of potential weakness, prone to damage by excessive shear forces as often occurs in the aetiology of pressure ulceration.

The hypodermis

This layer is composed of areola and adipose tissue. It also contains major blood vessels.
So that the many layers of the skin do not separate out, fibres extend down from the dermis into the hypodermis ensuring adhesion. The hypodermis is itself firmly attached to deeper structures.

Functions of the skin

The skin performs seven main functions:

1. Regulation of body temperature
2. Protection
3. Sensation
4. Excretion
5. Immunity
6. Blood reservoir
7. Synthesis of vitamin D

The human body maintains its temperature at around 37° centigrade. Variation of even a few degrees either way causes discomfort and affects biochemical function. The skin plays a major role in regulating body temperature. As environmental temperature rises the blood vessels in the peripheries dilate giving us a red appearance. Heat is lost through radiation. We also begin to sweat. The evaporation of sweat from the skins surface has a cooling effect, which also helps to keep body temperature within an acceptable range. Conversely, in response to a reducing environmental temperature the production of sweat decreases and peripheral blood vessels begin to constrict, reducing blood flow through the skin. Insulation to the circulation is thereby improved, conserving heat.

The lifelong potential for the skin to repair and regenerate makes it a unique and extremely effective protective physical barrier. It is flexible, waterproof and fairly robust. Unlike inert materials, breaches to the skin's surface caused by trauma, simply heal over. The body is thereby protected from bacterial invasion and also, to some extent, from damage by radiation.

The skin supplies the body with a vast array of sensory information. Both pleasant and noxious stimuli caused by temperature, touch, pressure and pain are perceived by nerve endings and receptors in the skin and transmitted as neural impulses to the brain.

In addition to sweat and excess heat, the skin is also able to excrete other unwanted material, such as waste products of metabolism and other organic compounds.

The function of the skin in preventing bacterial invasion by providing a physical barrier is further enhanced by the presence within the epidermis of specialised cells, which recognise and destroy foreign invaders and degrade and remove dead and damaged tissue. These cells form the outer ring of the immune system. Among the most important of these are the macrophages (big eaters) and the lymphocytes. Their role is to deactivate and ingest unwanted cellular material.

Other cells are particularly responsible for regrowth and regeneration. Of these, an important one is the fibroblast, which secretes growth factors and matrix proteins. Growth factors control and modulate a whole range of activities occurring within the healing wound bed. Fibroblasts also secrete proteases, which degrade non-viable tissue. The healing wound also contains a number of biochemical mediators such as the cytokines (Hunt *et al*, 2000). Cytokines are important in the regulation of the healing processes as they can attract other cells to the wound (chemoattractant) and are responsible for switching on and off various cellular activities within it. For example, if the activity of protease is excessive, degradation of regenerating tissue occurs, inhibiting healing.

The skin below the epidermis is extremely vascular and serves as a reservoir for blood. The extensive network of vessels within the dermis carry an estimated 8–10% of the total blood flow in a resting adult.

Although adequate quantities of vitamin D can be obtained from a diet that is sufficiently rich in milk and milk products, it can also be synthesised in the skin in the presence of sunlight. This is of particular benefit within cultures where milk is not normally consumed beyond childhood or for those people who have a milk intolerance.

Types of wound healing

Wounds are often described as healing by primary or first intention or by second intention. These terms are attributed to the Greek philosopher and physician, Hippocrates (circa 460 BC), but are still used today.

First intention

In first or primary intention, wound edges are re-approximated by sutures or clips and therefore heal faster because cells have less distance to migrate (Haas, 1995).

Second intention

In wounds healing by second intention, no attempt is made to close the wound in any way and any cavity has to fill in with granulation tissue. This process consequently takes much longer to complete.

The four stages of wound healing

Wound healing is a process which begins with the initial damage or injury and continues to the point where the body has effected as much repair as it can. As explained in *Chapter 2*, many factors affect wound healing. In addition to external factors, the size and nature of the wound will also significantly impact on the way in which any particular wound heals. Nevertheless, in all wounds several distinct stages have been identified. These stages have been given a variety of names. Here they are described as:

- inflammation
- reconstruction
- proliferation
- maturation.

It is important to remember that these stages are not discrete sequential entities but may overlap one another: that one or more of the stages may be present in the same wound at the same time. In addition, although time frames are given, these should be regarded as variable, dependant on a whole raft of local and systemic factors.

Inflammation

Inflammation is a normal reaction to tissue trauma and occurs shortly after the event. It is an essential part of the healing process as it alerts and mobilises the body's defence forces to limit the damage and initiate repair. The signs of inflammation — redness, heat, pain and swelling — are also identical to the body's response to bacterial invasion. When inflammatory signs are noticed within a wound it is important for the practitioner to question whether the cause is due to tissue damage or to infection as different management strategies may be required.

Following cell damage histamine, which triggers vasodilation, is released from mast cells. Vasodilation increases blood flow to the affected area and increases capillary permeability. Leucocytes are then able to squeeze through the capillary walls into the area of damaged tissue. The first leucocyte to arrive at the wound is the neutrophil and they can be found on the scene within the hour. They arrive in large numbers and begin on the process, known as phagocytosis, of breaking down and removing debris and any opportunistic bacteria from the area.

The area appears red because of the increased blood flow and the extra activity gives off heat. With so many cells, carried in plasma now outside the circulation, swelling occurs. This puts the tissues under tension causing pain which is further exacerbated by inflammatory chemical agents.

Other defence cells called macrophages appear in the wound. They are larger than neutrophils and are able to phagocytose larger particles. Neutrophils can live for a few hours or a few days but are then phagocytosed by the macrophages.

Inflammation lasts around four to five days, but can be prolonged by infection or irritation. Under certain circumstances it can be absent. This can occur if the patient is severely debilitated. Inflammation can also be suppressed by certain drugs, eg. steroids and non-steroidal anti-inflammatories.

Reconstruction

Once debris removal has commenced, reconstruction can begin. Macrophages now produce growth factors which attract fibroblasts to the wound. Fibroblasts are the cells which produce collagen fibres, the basic building matrix upon which new tissue structures are built. A prime activity is the growth of new blood vessels in the area, which carry oxygen and nutrients to the wound. These new vessels loop in and around the collagen matrix to form a network. The buds of sprouting new blood vessels appear knobbly or granular, the basis of granulation tissue. Collagen has been seen in a new wound as early as the second day.

Some specialised fibroblasts known as myofibroblasts have a further role. They have a contractile apparatus which causes the wound to shrink by pulling the edges together. That is why even very large wounds may contract down to leave a fairly modest scar. This shrinkage may start about the fifth or sixth day and it has been estimated that contraction may account for as much as 40% of wound closure (Haas, 1995).

The time required for reconstruction will depend on many factors such as initial wound size and degree of damage and anatomical location.

Proliferation

This phase occurs when the wound bed has filled in sufficiently for the epithelium to grow over and, dependant on the depth of the defect, can begin within hours after injury. Epithelial cells can only grow across the wound from the edge or from remnants of epithelial structures, eg. hair follicles or sweat glands still present in the wound bed.

These cells migrate from the wound margins, moving across one another in a leapfrog fashion. When cells meet in the centre of the wound or at the edges, they stop proliferating. This is known as contact inhibition.

These cells can only move over viable tissue and require a moist environment so that if they meet an eschar (a hard dry structure commonly called a scab) they will burrow under it (Haas, 1995).

Maturation

Long after the functional barrier of the skin has been restored, the maturation process will continue. Collagen continues to be deposited but, even at one year, wound strength is never more than 80% of what it once was and never totally regains its pre-injury tensile state (Haas, 1995).

As maturation continues, because there is no longer the need to bring new cells into the area, a reduction in vascularity occurs and the scar tissue becomes less red in colour. Scarring also becomes flatter and more comparable to normal tissue.

Key points

❖ The skin is a strong, durable, renewable, multilayer structure, which has seven discrete functions.

❖ Wound healing is a complex process, which is still not fully understood.

❖ There are four overlapping stages of wound healing and wounds can be said to heal by primary or secondary intention.

❖ A basic knowledge of the physiology of the skin and the wound healing process is essential for effective wound management.

References

Brooker C (1993) *Human Structure and Function*. 2nd edn. Mosby, London

Haas A (1995) Wound healing. *Dermatology Nurs* **7**(1): 28–34, 74

Hunt TK, Hopf H, Hussain Z (2000) Physiology of wound healing. *Adv Skin Wound Care* **13**(6): 6

Chapter 2

Wound assessment

This chapter will examine and describe the various factors that need consideration when assessing wounds. These factors will include examination of the patient and their lifestyle, together with their health status.

The need for assessment

Accurate wound assessment forms the basis of any clinical decision making and is a sound investment in time. Effective wound management depends on the appropriate selection of dressings and treatments, which can only be determined by a thorough and knowledgeable wound assessment. It is also a fascinating subject – the more you know, the more you can identify and the better your decision-making skills become.

Many patients have their wounds managed without any formal wound assessment. The wound management products may have been chosen for the following reasons:

- they were available in the dressings cupboard
- they were the same product used last time
- you really like a particular product and tend to use it a great deal.

Reflective activity

Consider some of the patients with wounds you have managed in the past. How did you reach your clinical decisions? Were any of the above statements true for you?

In these situations, the products are not chosen to meet the individual needs of the patient and there is no guarantee that they are receiving the best possible care.

Another important reason for having an accurate assessment is to improve documentation and communication. Statements such as 'healing well' are actually quite meaningless. The United Kingdom Central Council for Nursing, Midwifery and Health Visiting (UKCC, now the Nursing and Midwifery Council [NMC]) in its guidelines for records and record keeping (1998), states that good record keeping helps to protect the patients and clients by promoting:

- High standards of clinical care.
- Continuity of care.
- Better communication and dissemination of information between members and the inter-professional team.
- An accurate account of treatment and care planning and delivery.
- The ability to detect problems, such as changes in the patient's condition at an early stage.

In the event of any complaint, nursing records are one of the first sources to be investigated and so it is important that they should be as accurate as possible. Patients have a legal right to see them too.

A sound baseline assessment is important to evaluate subsequent healing or deterioration of the wound. It will also enable the tissue viability practitioner to judge how successful the treatment plan and choice of wound dressings has been.

Patient considerations

None of us can actually heal wounds – we can only provide the optimum conditions for the patient to heal himself or herself. This is why it is important to consider the patient before embarking on any wound management plan. The following will need careful consideration.

General physical condition

The overall health of the patient will have the strongest influence on how a wound heals. In terms of disease processes, any condition that reduces the supply of oxygen to the wound, such as cardiac disease, anaemia or chronic breathing difficulties are likely to delay healing (Miller, 1999). Smoking also limits the amount of oxygen available for wound healing (Siana and Gottrup, 1992). Any form of substance abuse, including alcohol, will have a detrimental effect on wound healing. Flanagan (1997) enlarges upon this with the following table (*Table 2.1*).

Table 2.1: Conditions that prolong healing	
Circulatory disorders	Malabsorption disorders
• anaemia	• Chrohn's disease
• peripheral vascular disease	• ulcerative collitis
• arteriosclerosis	
Respiratory disorders	Disorders of mobility and sensation
• chronic obstructive airway disease	• Cerebral vascular accident (CVA)
• bronchitis	• spinal injury
• pneumonia	• neuropathy
Metabolic disorders	Immune deficiency disorders
• diabetes	• rheumatoid arthritis
• renal and hepatic failure	• HIV, AIDS
	• malignancy

Nutrition

Any deficiencies in the amount and quality of nutrients will prolong the healing process, and may result in complications. The risk of developing pressure ulceration also increases.

The generation of new tissue in the process of wound healing is a demanding activity on the body's reserves. The greater the extent of the injury, the more energy will be required.

The main energy source for all the activities is from glucose that may be required in increased amounts. Dietary protein is required for a number of cellular functions including the synthesis of enzymes, antibodies and some hormones. Protein deficiencies can result in prolonged inflammatory process, decreased collagen synthesis and an increased risk of wound dehiscence (Lewis, 1996; Russell, 2001). Vitamins, trace elements and amino acids play an important role in collagen synthesis, wound tensile strength, blood clotting and in the fight against infection. These too may be required in increased amounts. Important nutrients include vitamins C, A, B and K, zinc, copper and iron (Lewis, 1996).

People at risk from poor nutrition include those with a decreased appetite, those who have undergone major surgery or those who have a high exudate loss (eg. through a fistula). Patients aged over sixty-five years of age, who have a body mass index (BMI) less than 24 kg/m^2 or those who have lost 5% or more of their body weight in the previous one to two months, have been shown to be at significant nutritional risk (Beck and Ovesen, 1998).

A thorough nutritional assessment will need to be carried out. This should include careful observation and recording of what the patient actually eats. This information will then allow analysis of protein, vitamin and mineral as well as calorific intake. Weight loss will be detected by regularly weighing the patient. These measurements, combined with the height of the patient will also allow calculation of body mass index which is a height for weight ratio.

Dehydration can also have a negative effect on wound healing and can result in electrolyte imbalance. Fluid and nutritional loss may increase in patients who have heavily exuding wounds or fistulas.

Reflective activity

Consider a patient from your own practice who presented with a wound healing via secondary intention. List the number of ways in which nutrition needs were assessed and addressed. On reflection, do you consider these to have been adequate? How could they have been improved?

Psychosocial

It is important to consider how the presence of the wound and resulting treatment may be affecting the patient and how it is disrupting their normal lifestyle. Factors such as attending clinics, waiting in for the district nurse or having to cope with treatments such as compression bandaging can be perceived as stressful. The presence of a wound may have resulted in a negative body image for the patient. A study by Kiecolt–Glaser *et al* (1995) demonstrated how stress can delay healing in healthy volunteers. Fully involving patients in each aspect of their care may help to encourage a feeling of control over their situation.

Other considerations

⌘ Care situation – who is caring for the patient and what are the available facilities and level of expertise?

⌘ Understanding and compliance — if the patient is made aware of your treatment aims and reasoning behind them then you are more likely to have a patient who will work with you. This is important when treatments such as compression bandaging are necessary. It may also help to overcome anxiety and stress for your patient as these have been shown to have negative effects on all aspects of health.

⌘ Medication — some medications, such as; steroids, immunosuppressive agents, anti-coagulants or cytotoxic drugs will have a negative effect on wound healing and must be considered.

⌘ The age of the patient will influence their ability to heal as the repair process slows down with age. Cells such as fibroblasts which synthesis collagen and macrophages decrease in number and epithelialisation is slower. The skin itself changes with reduced collagen and elastin. There is also a flattening of the dermo-epidermal junction (where the two layers join) which results in more fragile tissue that is less resistant to shearing forces such as pressure ulceration (Desai, 1997; Miller, 1999).

Patient scenario one

Mr Frank Skelton is an eighty-two-year-old widower who was admitted to your hospital two weeks ago following a stroke. He had collapsed at home one morning in his bedroom while attempting to get to the toilet. He was found propped up in the corner of the bedroom by his neighbour later that morning. However it was several hours before he could be persuaded to go into hospital by ambulance.

Within a few days of his admission, a large sacral pressure ulcer was noted.

Assessment and biochemistry found him to be anaemic and in a poor nutritional state. He has smoked since his youth and continues to smoke approximately ten cigarettes a day. He suffers from chronic bronchitis, particularly in the winter months.

His prescribed medication on admission was frusemide, arthrotec and ferrous sulphate. He stated that he was allergic to penicillin.

Mr Skelton found that his pressure ulcer ached from time to time and that he found dressing changes to be painful and distressing.

He is responding well to his rehabilitation programme but, as yet, is unable to walk without the assistance of two helpers.

Activity one

List six factors from your general nursing assessment that are of relevance and interest to the tissue viability status of Mr Skelton.

1.

2.

3.

4.

5.

6.

Looking at the wound

Your aim, when looking at the wound, should be to gather a wide range of data which you can use to evaluate the situation and plan your care. This will require clearly defined goals which are realistic to your patient's situation and your own. For example, consider the problems in managing a community-based patient with a wet, exuding wound. Nursing staff may not be readily available if the dressing was not able to contain the exudate for an acceptable period of time.

Your assessments should be ongoing so that you can gauge how effective your care has been. Involving your patient and their carers in this can help to motivate them. As a general rule, wounds should be reassessed weekly unless there is a change in the condition of the wound or in the patients themselves.

What do you need to know when assessing a wound?

The first step in wound assessment is to classify the wound using the following criteria.

Cause of wound

The history and appearance of the wound can determine this information. It is important to have an understanding of the causal pathophysiology of different wounds (such as the ulceration that occurs as a result of chronic venous hypertension) in order to treat the cause as well as the wound itself.

Duration of wound

An acute wound is one that progresses through the normal stages of healing within an acceptable time frame and without complications, eg. sutured surgical wounds, lacerations, abrasions. An acute wound that does not heal within an expected time frame will require further investigation to determine the factors responsible for the extended healing time (Flanagan, 1997).

A chronic wound, on the other hand, has been defined as a wound that fails to heal as anticipated or that has been stuck in any one phase of wound healing for a period of six weeks or more (Collier, 2003). It does not proceed to full healing. Examples of these are pressure ulcers and leg ulcers. They usually become stuck in the inflammatory phase of healing and tend to produce lots of exudate. Control of this exudate is vital if these wounds are to go on to full healing.

Depth of wound

Superficial wounds involve loss of epidermal cells while partial-thickness wounds also include the dermis. In most cases they will heal by wound contraction.

Full-thickness wounds involve complete loss of both the epidermis and dermis, the subcutaneous tissue or even deeper structures, such as muscle and bone may be visible. Tendons and ligaments may also be present, as in the case of full depth pressure ulceration to the heel. If there is a lot of wound debris present, it may not be possible to judge how deep the wound is. If there is a track or sinus present and you can not see the end, the wound should be classified as full-thickness (see following section for more information on tracks and sinuses).

Site of wound

This may have implications for dressing fixation as areas such as the sacrum, scalp and heels are difficult to dress. The site of the wound can also reveal a great deal about the cause of the wound. An ulcer in the gaiter region of the lower leg is probably venous in origin (Young, 1997).

Stage of healing

Different tissue types and exudate levels will be apparent for the different phases of healing. For example, a wound in the inflammatory phase may have slough and necrotic tissue present with lots of exudate. The white cells and proteolyic enzymes present in the exudate will be working to remove the slough and necrosis.

Tissue type

It is important to determine the different tissue within a wound. Many wounds, especially if chronic, will contain a mixture.

There is no standard method of describing tissue types. Colour coding is often used which is simple and easy, however, there may be problems with interpreting colour. Descriptive terms can also be used which require a greater knowledge base.

The various tissue types are as follows and are illustrated in *Figures 2.1–2.5*.

❖ *Epithelial tissue (pink)*

This tissue is present in the final stages of healing as it forms the new epidermis. Epithelial cells migrate from the wound margins or from hair follicles and sweat glands in partial-thickness wounds (this appears as small white islands within the wound and are often seen in venous leg ulcers).

❖ *Granulation tissue (red)*

This tissue is bright red in appearance and is very moist. Its function is to replace any lost dermis and to fill any defect. It can become raised (over-granulation), although this is usually self-limiting. Unhealthy granulation tissue that is dark and dull in appearance and that bleeds easily may be infected (Cutting and Harding, 1994).

❖ *Slough (yellow)*

Slough consists of dead cells and wound debris and is usually yellow in appearance. It varies in consistency from thick and fibrous (usually found in the base of chronic wounds) to thin, watery and fibrinous (this is often found when the connective tissue matrix is being laid down in preparation for granulation tissue). Some wounds, such as venous leg ulcers, tend to be covered in a layer of superficial slough.

❖ *Necrotic tissue (black)*

Necrotic tissue is dead tissue and may appear as black, brown or (when hydrated) grey material within a wound. Dehydrated necrotic tissue is often referred to as eschar. As this tissue is devitalised it cannot regenerate and must be removed. Its presence inhibits wound healing and provides a breeding area for micro-organisms. It may well obscure the actual wound bed making accurate wound assessment impossible; black heels are a good example of this. Necrosis can also occur in patches within a wound usually combined with slough.

❖ *Infected tissue (green)*

Careful observation is needed to assess for the possibility of wound infection. This process elicits a marked host immune response (Mertz and Ovington, 1993). These responses are visible as clinical signs and include: localised heat, pain, swelling and erythema. There may well be a purulent discharge, uncharacteristic odour and increased pain. The patient may also feel unwell and have a raised or even lowered body temperature. Additional criteria also need consideration. Cutting and Harding (1994) suggest the following:

- dark, weak friable granulation tissue that bleeds easily
- pitting at the base of the wound
- bridging of weak epithelial tissue
- wounds that do not heal when all other factors have been considered.

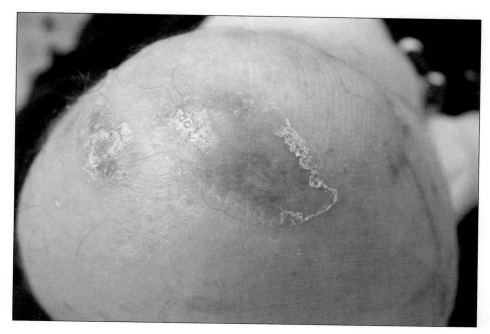

Figure 2.3: Epithelial tissue

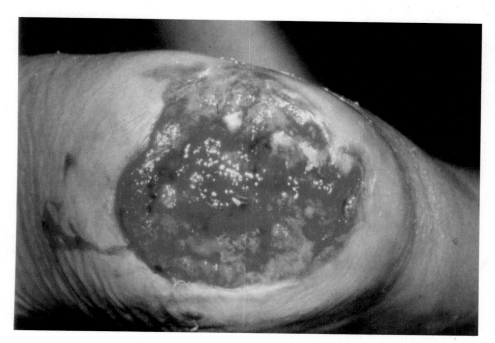

Figure 2.1: Granulation tissue

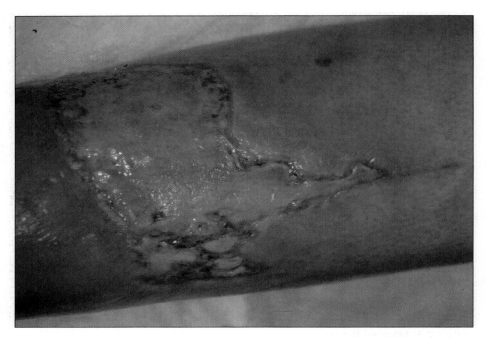

Figure 2.2: Slough

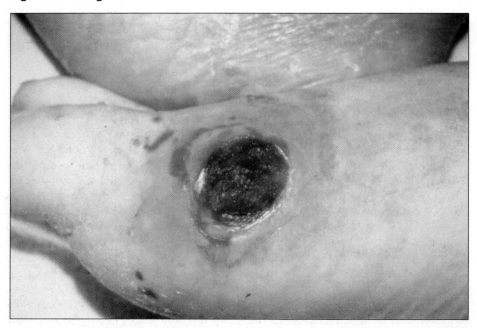

Figure 2.4: Necrotic tissue

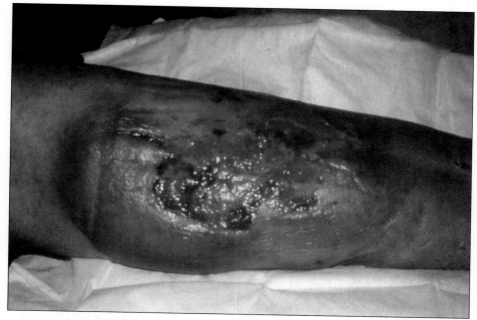

Figure 2.5: Infected tissue

The elderly and immunocompromised patients may not exhibit easily detectable clinical signs of infection (Kiernan, 1997). The colour coding of green for an infected wound can be misleading. A wound that is colonised with a green staining organism such as *Psuedomonas aeruginosa* may not necessarily be infected.

Identifying infection

When clinical signs of infection are present, a wound swab is normally taken in order to identify the causative organism. The reliability of this method of sampling has been questionned (Kelly, 2003) and there is little consensus agreement on how best to take swabs (Gilchrist, 1996). The recommended technique is to rotate the swab between the fingers while sampling the wound using a zigzag motion. This allows you to cover a greater area of both the swab and the wound. It is important that you send a bacterial sample and not one that just contains dressing debris. For this reason it may be best to clean the wound first if any debris is present. Always put as much information as you can for the laboratory staff. If the presence of necrosis and malodour is mentioned, this will alert them to check for anaerobes (such as bacteroides or clostridium). If there is pus present a sample should be sent off for analysis instead. Always check the results and do not be afraid of contacting the lab is you are unsure about them. If antibiotic sensitivities are given on the result form, they should only be prescribed if the signs of infection persist. It must be remembered that wound swabs will only detect bacteria from the surface of the wound (Gilchrist, 1996). The results can give a false positive, where the isolated surface bacteria is not causing the infection. A false negative result will occur if the causative bacteria is not isolated from the swab (it may be found only in the deeper tissues).

Cellulitis

In addition to wound infection, areas of skin and subcutaneous tissue may also become invaded by bacteria. This condition is known as cellulitis and is often linked to two main organisms *Staphlococcus aureus* and *ß-haemolytic Streptoccocus* (Baxter and McGregor, 2001). Sometimes no predisposing cause can be found but usually some insult which has provided a portal of entry for the micro-organisms can be found. Risk factors include diabetes and oedema, peripheral vascular disease and presence of fungal infection, eg. tinea pedis (www.jbmedical.com/cellulitisbackground 2003). The patient may well present with the usual signs and symptoms of infection but lymphangitis, lymphadenopathy, rigors and malaise may also be present. The condition is serious and medical help should be sought immediately. Often it is difficult, if not impossible, to isolate the offending organism through blood culture (Baxter and McGregor, 2001) other blood investigations may well give a raised white cell and C-reactive protein count. The standard treatment is oral antibiotics together with rest, analgesia and elevation of the affected part (if applicable).

> *Time out*
>
> Look at the wounds shown in *Figures 2.1–2.5*. Using the above descriptions of tissue type estimate the percentage coverage for each tissue type.

Condition of surrounding skin

The presence of any erythema or cellulitis should be noted as both these indicate the presence of inflammation or infection. Maceration of surrounding tissue will result from prolonged exposure to moisture. Skin conditions such as eczema and dry, flaky skin can result in additional distress for the patient. Problems can arise from the use of wound management products themselves. Trauma to the skin can arise from frequent and inappropriate removal of adhesive dressings while some patients may develop a contact dermatitis to the dressings, products and tapes (Dealey, 1999).

Wound edge

A healthy wound edge will allow the migration of new epidermal cells. In certain cases the wound edge can become altered and healing may not be able to progress. In some chronic wounds, there may be undermining of the wound edge in that it extends under the top layer of skin. Any abnormal, raised wound edges should be referred for further investigation, as they could be indicative of malignancy.

Exudate level

The amount of exudate present in each wound will be influenced by a number of factors. Exudate plays an important role in the inflammatory stage of wound healing and is produced in significant amounts. The growth factors and proteolytic enzymes contained within the exudate are required for clearing wound debris and for stimulating cells necessary for advancing the healing process. Oedema, hydrostatic pressure, infection, or foreign bodies such as dressing debris, will all influence the amount of exudate present in a wound.

Exudate is normally pale amber in colour but may become discoloured in the presence of infection (yellow, green), while trauma may cause it to become blood stained (Young, 2000). Exudate from chronic wounds has been found to be different in nature to that found in acute wounds. Studies have shown that chronic wound exudate contains high levels of proteolytic enzymes (Hart, 2002; Philips *et al*, 1998. Parnham, 2002). These degrade fibronectin that is a key component of the wound matrix or scaffolding that is laid down to support the new tissue. Many chronic wounds such as leg ulcers are highly exuding. It is easy to see why a vicious cycle of building up and breaking down new wound structures can occur. Heavy exudate loss will also effect the nutritional status of the patient, as considerable amounts of protein can be lost in this way. Assessment of the amount of exudate present is subjective, and should take into consideration the amount, colour and consistency (Young, 1997). The terms low, moderate or heavy are often used to describe the amount of exudate. Monitoring the length of time a dressing can remain *in situ* without strike through will provide valuable information on the amount of exudate being produced.

Although the aim is to provide a moist environment for the wound, too much exudate can cause maceration and excoriation of the skin and will result in frequent dressing changes. Exudate that is not contained by dressings and leaks through onto clothes will have a detrimental effect on the patient. It could lead to social isolation, withdrawal and despondency.

Pain

Pain can have a detrimental effect on the patient and can adversely influence the entire healthcare experience. Effective assessment and management of pain is vital to any wound management plan. Assessment should begin by talking to the patient about their pain and by observing any responses. This subject is discussed in more detail in the following chapter (*pp. 26–29*).

Odour

Wounds become malodorous when there are either specific or excessive amounts of bacteria in the wound. The presence of necrotic tissue will also influence odour, as it will provide an ideal environment for bacteria. Certain dressing materials, such as hydrocolloids, can give a distinctive odour on removal. Malodour can have a negative effect on patients and can result in social isolation. The measurement of odour is subjective and the patient's perception should always be considered as it may be different to your own. Efforts should always be taken to eliminate odour as quickly as possible, either by treatment of infection or use of odour reducing dressings, such as charcoal.

Ability of dressings to cope with wound condition

Your assessment should also extend to the dressings and any fixatives such as tapes. The following questions will help determine the effectiveness of your chosen dressing:

⌘ Is there evidence of dressing 'strike through' or any damage to skin (the chosen dressing may be unable to cope with the level of exudate or its wear-time has been too long)?

⌘ Is the dressing intact and firmly attached to the skin (if not leakage and soiling can occur)?

⌘ Is the dressing comfortable and not causing any rubbing and irritation?

⌘ Is the dressing visible under clothing?

⌘ Has the dressing interfered with function in any way?

There are some situations, such as in the care of a fungating, malignant wound, where wound healing is not likely to be achieved. In these instances, the performance and exudate handling properties of any wound product becomes a major priority. Further information on the selection of dressings is provided in *Chapter 3*.

Wound assessment charts

These are often used to assist with documentation and should be used as an integral part of the care plan. They should incorporate sufficient room for more in-depth descriptions if needed and should incorporate a standardised language and use of descriptive terms (Hon and Jones, 2003). The wound assessment chart and care plan should also specify method of wound cleansing, frequency of dressing changes, pain management and other specific requirements pertinent to the patient. An example of a wound assessment chart is included in *Appendix 1*.

Descriptive terminology

Knowledge of anatomy and anatomical terminology can assist in describing the position of wounds more accurately. The following reference planes and descriptive terms are useful for wound descriptions and should form part of a common language to be used when describing wounds (Nelson, 2000):

⌘ The coronal plane divides the body into front and back. Structures to the front of the body are described as anterior while those to the back are posterior.

⌘ The median or sagittal plane divides the body into left and right. Structures near this line are medial while those further away are lateral.

⌘ The point of attachment of any limb (shoulder, hip) is used as reference points. Anything near these points would be proximal while anything further away would be distal.

⌘ The palms of the hands and soles of the feet are described as palmar and plantar and the opposite side is referred to as the dorsal surface.

Measuring wounds

Measuring the size and depth of a wound is important but is often overlooked. It is a vital part of a baseline assessment as this information is required to judge if your interventions have been successful or not. Ideally, measurements should be undertaken and recorded on a weekly basis. The following are all methods you can use.

Measuring and tracing

The use of a ruler or measuring scale will allow you to measure simple dimensions of a wound. Disposable paper scales or metal or plastic rulers that can be properly cleaned or sterilised afterwards will reduce the risk of spreading infection. Tracing sheets are a better option, particularly the ones that have two layers. The layer placed next to the wound can then be disposed of, leaving the top, uncontaminated layer, for your records. They do have a tendency of misting up when placed on the wound, which can make recording details difficult. You can calculate the surface area by adding up all the full squares that fall within the wound. Half squares can be added up in the same way to give a total figure (Flanagan, 1997). If you do not have access to these, a simple disposable, sterile glove can be used in the same way.

It is important to put in as much information as you can, such as demarcation lines for tissue types and any surrounding areas of erythema. Always remember to orientate the tracings by adding body landmarks, eg. arrow toward the head. These methods will provide you with a rough estimate of size, however, this will only be two-dimensional and little information will be gained about the wound bed. Wounds on curved surfaces or awkward areas such as heels, elbows and the axilla will prove difficult to measure using these methods.

Photographing wounds

This is the better option, especially if undertaken by a medical photographer. A photographic image will greatly enhance any record on wound healing and can be valuable if the patient is moved to another healthcare setting during the wound-healing episode.

If you are taking a series of photos always try and take them from the same distance and angle and to incorporate the same background. The use of a measuring scale will assist in measuring the size. The advent of digital cameras has made photography simpler and it is also possible for the patients to view their wounds using the small image-viewing screen. This is a great method of involving the patient. Consent needs to be gained prior to photographing any wound, and consideration given to secure storage to comply with the data protection requirements. Photographs should not include the patient's face for confidentiality reasons. Computerised measuring programmes are now available which can work in conjunction with digital images to provide an accurate surface area measurement.

Measuring depth

Three-dimensional measurements are required for deeper wounds. Measurements of depth can be made using gloved fingers, probes or sterile single use urinary catheters. It is important that you do not damage tissue when doing this or hurt the patient. These measurements are not accurate and can underestimate the size.

Sinuses and areas of undermining are more difficult to measure. A sinogram can provide more accurate information. This procedure involves injecting radio-opaque dye into the wound.

It is useful to describe the direction of any sinus' and areas of undermining using a clock face (the patient's head would be at 12 o'clock) (Flanagan, 1997). Another method is to draw on the skin the corresponding area of undermining which can be determined by gentle examination using a probe.

Conditions requiring specialist referral

There are a number of situations within wound care that require specialist input to eliminate the presence of underlying conditions, such as vascular disease, dermatological conditions or malignancy. The following are examples of situations when further advice from an appropriate practition should be sought:

- if the wound fails to heal despite thorough assessment and best practice
- any unexplained deterioration in the wound condition, including colour and odour.
- change in pain status, or pain that would seem to be inappropriate for the wound
- any unusual presentation within the wound or of the wound edge
- any wound that presents where the cause is unknown
- any evidence of self-harm or non-accidental injury.

Patient scenario two

Mr Skelton and his presenting pressure ulcer are shown in *Figures 2.6* and *2.7*. Undertake a general wound assessment of his pressure ulcer by using either the wound assessment chart included in the appendices or a chart from your own clinical area. Include two-dimensional measurements.

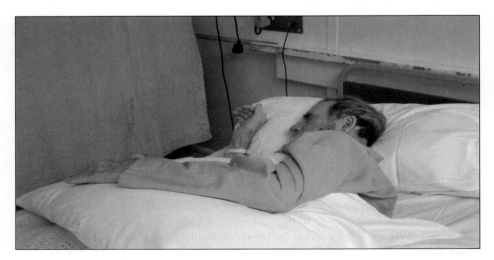

Figure 2.6: Mr Skelton (patient scenario)

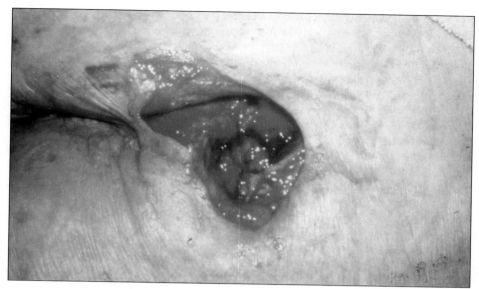

Figure 2.7: Mr Skelton's pressure ulcer

Key points

❖ Accurate wound assessment forms the basis of any clinical decision making. It is required in order to evaluate subsequent healing or deterioration of the wound and to improve both documentation and communication with other members of the healthcare team.

❖ The patients' condition must be considered before embarking on any plan of care. This will include general physical health, nutrition, age, medication, care situation and psychosocial considerations.

❖ Observational skills are critical when assessing wounds. Information will be required not only on the cause and duration but also on the tissue type, condition of the surrounding skin and factors such as pain, odour and exudate levels.

❖ Measuring the size and depth of a wound is important but is often overlooked. This can be achieved by a number of methods including measuring and tracing and photography.

References

Baxter H, McGregor F (2001) Understanding and managing. *Cellulitis* **15**(44): 50–6

Beck AM, Ovesen L (1998) At which body mass index and degree of weight loss should hospitalised elderly patients should be considered at nutritional risk? *Clinical Nutrition* **17**: 195–8

Collier, M (2003) Wound bed preparation: theory to practice. *Nurs Standard* **17**(36): 45–55

Cutting K, Harding K (1994) Criteria for identifying wound infection. *J Wound Care* **3**(4): 198–201

Dealey C (1999) *The Care of Wounds: A guide for nurses.* Blackwell Science, Oxford

Desai H (1997) Ageing and wounds Part 2; healing in old age. *J Wound Care* **6**(5): 237–9

Field L, Adams N (2001) Pain management 2: the use of psychological approaches to pain. *Br J Nurs* **10**(15): 971–4

Flanagan M (1997) Wound assessment. In: Flanagan M, ed. *Wound Management.* Churchill Livingstone, London

Gilchrist B (1996) Wound infection: Sampling bacterial flora: a review of the literature. *J Wound Care* **5**: 386–8

Hart J (2002) Inflammation 2; its role in the healing of chronic wounds. *J Wound Care* **11**(7): 245–9

Hon J, Jones C (2003) The documentation of wounds in an acute hospital setting. *Br J Nurs* **5**(17): 1040–5

Kelly F (2003) Infection control: validity and reliability in wound swabbing. *Br J Nurs* **12**(16): 959–64

Kiecolt-Glaser JK, Maruncvha P, Malarkey W, Mercado A, Glaser W (1995) Slowing of wound healing by psychological stress. *Lancet* **346**: 11946

Kiernan M (1997) Infected wounds: diagnosis and treatment. *Practice Nurs* **8**(13): 39–42

Lewis B (1996) Nutritional intake and the risk of pressure sore development in older patients. *J Wound Care* **7**(1): 31–5

Mertz PM, Ovington LG (1993) Wound healing microbiology. *Dermatalogic Clinics* **11**(4): 739–47

Miller M (1999) Wound assessment. In: *Wound Management, Theory and Practice.* Nursing Times books, EMAP healthcare, London

elson A (2000) Accurate documentation. *Nurs Times Plus* **96**(4) 10–11

Parnham A (2002) Moist wound healing: does the theory apply to chronic wounds? *J Wound Care* **11**(4): 143–6

Phillips T, Al-Amoundi H, Leverkus M, Park H-Y (1998) Effects of chronic wound fluid on fibroblasts. *J Wound Care* **7**(10): 527–32

Russell L (2001) The importance of patients' nutritional status in wound healing. *Br J Nurs* (Supplement) **10**(6): S42–S49

Siana JE, Gottrup F (1992) The effects of smoking on tissue function. *J Wound Care* **1**(2): 37–41

United Kingdom Central Council for Nursing, Midwifery and Health Visiting (1998) *Guidelines for Records and Record Keeping.* UKCC, London

Young T (1997) Wound assessment and documentation. *Practice Nurs* **8**(13): 27–30

Young T (2000) Managing exudate. *Essential Wound Healing Bulletin.* Part 6, EMAP Healthcare, London

Chapter 3

Wound healing therapies

Wound bed preparation

Definition

Wound healing depends on many diverse factors, not least the general health, well-being and social environment in which the patient lives. It also depends on the correct management of the wound itself. When a practitioner first encounters a wound there may be a number of local factors to be addressed before that wound has arrived at a state in which healing can take place. That initial process is called wound bed preparation.

Wound bed preparation has been defined as, 'the management of a wound in order to accelerate endogenous healing or to facilitate the effectiveness of other therapeutic measures' (Schultz *et al*, 2003). The aim being to create an optimal wound healing environment which is stable, well vascularised and with minimal exudate (Dowsett, 2002). To achieve this aim practitioners require an adequate understanding of what the healing wound needs and how to provide it.

Key components

Five key components of wound bed preparation have been identified (Dowsett, 2002):

- management of necrosis
- management of wound exudate
- restoring bacterial balance
- correcting cellular dysfunction
- restoring biochemical balance.

Debridement

Necrosis may be removed in several ways. Surgical and sharp debridement are methods by which the dead tissue is cut away. It is cheap, quick and effective but should only be undertaken by appropriately trained practitioners. Autolysis is the means by which the body's own defence mechanism produces enzymes which break down and remove necrotic tissue. This process is much slower, but if the amount is small and the wound is kept moist it will be successful. A quicker method is the use of larval therapy (*Chapter 5*). One particular benefit of this method is that larvae can be used in areas where sharp or surgical debridement would be unsafe, eg. where other structures such as tendons are visible within the wound.

Moisture level

It has long been known that wounds heal best given a moist rather than a dry environment (Winter, 1962), but moist means moist, not wet. An excess of exudate within a wound can also inhibit healing (Ennis and Meneses, 2000). Control of exudate is essential. This is usually achieved by selecting a dressing of the appropriate absorbency. If exudate levels are particularly high, vacuum therapy may be an appropriate alternative (*Chapter 5*, 'Alternative, specialist and advanced therapies').

Bacterial load

The bacterial load of a wound will depend on several factors. Acute wounds host similar microorganisms to those found on intact skin whereas chronic wounds will host a much wider and greater range of bacteria (Mertz and Ovington, 1993). All wounds contain some microorganisms: their presence within a wound alone does not by itself constitute a wound infection. The relationship between bacterial numbers and the strength of the host response has been described as having three main stages:

- contamination
- colonisation
- infection.

Contamination is when small numbers of bacteria may be detected in a wound but their presence is transient and they are not multiplying.

In the colonised wound, however, the levels of organisms have not only increased but they have become established (Cooper and Lawrence, 1996). An intermediate stage between colonisation and infection is also sometimes referred to as critical colonisation. This is the stage where there is a heavy bacterial load, especially of certain types of organisms, which may delay healing (Mertz and Ovington,1993).

True clinical infection is defined as the process by which organisms bind to, multiply and then invade viable tissue. Managing infection within a wound does depend on identifying the responsible organism so that the correct systemic antibiotic therapy can commence as soon as possible. Other measures for reducing bacterial load include the removal of necrotic tissue and slough, which can harbour bacteria, the control of excess exudate and the selection of an appropriate dressing.

Once a wound is sustained a whole series of triggered events occur, known as the healing cascade. In optimum health and given optimum conditions wounds heal uneventfully, but sometimes a wound fails to make progress and becomes chronic. In the case of venous leg ulceration, the application of the appropriate compression can reactivate the wound and stimulate healing. Surgical debridement, because it takes the wound back to an earlier stage in the healing process, may likewise reactivate the healing cascade. A whole new range of products, which may be regarded as treatments rather than dressings, are becoming available to address the problem of the static wound. These products include growth factors and protease inhibitors (Collier, 2003).

The purpose of these products is to provide the missing link in the chain, so that the wound, which is failing to make expected progress, may go on to heal. These issues are discussed more fully in *Chapter 5* ('Tissue engineering', *p. 88*). Currently, determining what, if anything, is missing from a wound is not easily assessed. The practitioner must rely on more established but less direct methods such as blood biochemistry and wound bed biopsy to gain further information.

Wound cleansing

Wound cleansing is a subject over which there has been much debate. Issues have included when to cleanse, how to cleanse and with what. Arguments as to the rights and wrongs of using antibacterial cleansers have been heated and longstanding (Brennan, 1985; Lawrence, 1996). Methods of cleansing include irrigation, swabbing and bathing or showering, with controversy over the safety of the latter and over the correct pressures to apply during irrigation (Oliver,1997).

If cleansing is not viewed as part of wound bed preparation it can become a separate, somewhat ritualistic, activity performed for its own sake. Applied practically, it means only cleansing the wound if doing so will further the five key components of wound bed preparation. As Hippocrates is reported to have said, 'do no harm!' Strategy should be based on providing minimal necessary intervention, not adding anything the wound doesn't need and not taking away anything that it does. The following are general suggestions:

⌘ If there is necrotic tissue, soiling, old dressing remains, dried or excessive exudate, debris or other potential irritant substance present, then work to remove it.

⌘ Any cleansing method should seek to avoid unnecessary trauma. Damage to capillary beds causing bleeding will elicit a fresh inflammatory response. Use swabs judiciously. At times they may be necessary but swabbing can result in fibres being left in the wound which can also delay healing (Wood, 1976).

⌘ Solutions used should be non-irritant and free of bacteria. Normal saline is the most commonly used wound cleanser but in large quantities this may not be practicable. A community study found no difference in infection and healing rates when tap water was used (Griffiths *et al*, 2001).

⌘ Mitotic activity (cell division in the healing wound) occurs optimally at 37°C with cooled wounds taking several hours to regain their previous state (Lock, 1980). Use solutions to body temperature.

⌘ If the wound is clean, healthy, granulating and happy it does not require cleansing and to do so may disturb the normal healing wound environment.

⌘ Don't use swabs routinely to dry the wound bed, as it needs to stay moist. However, the surrounding healthy skin must be dried well to avoid maceration and to facilitate the fixation of adhesive dressings and tape.

⌘ Use a cleansing method appropriate for the wound. Irrigation of a discharging tracheostomy wound with a syringe could result in inhalation of the irrigant. Swabbing, in this instance, is likely to be the best method. Whereas trying to swab bilateral leg ulcers would be at best time-consuming and possibly ineffective. They would perhaps be best managed in a bucket kept for that purpose, lined with a clean plastic bag.

⌘ Anti-bacterials and other cleansing agents are still used in some areas under certain circumstances. The practitioner using them needs to be aware of the reasons for this, the safety of the practice and the correct dilution, duration of contact and method of application.

Pain

Pain is a complex and subjective sensation that is influenced by many factors. The results of a recent international study (Moffatt *et al*, 2003) demonstrated that dressing removal is considered to be the time of most pain and that dried out dressings and adherent products are most likely to cause pain and trauma at dressing changes. Patients who have been subjected to painful dressing changes may remember this experience and become anxious at the prospect of further experiences. Health-related quality of life studies have shown that pain improves significantly with effective treatment that prevents healing. Assessment should begin by talking to the patient about their pain and by observing any responses. The use of a validated visual analogue scale can established the severity of the pain (Briggs *et al*, 2003). Strategies for eliminating wound pain include the use of appropriate analgesia giving at the correct time; careful dressing selection and time spent talking to the patient to reduce their anxieties. Adequate knowledge of the wound and its subsequent management can enhance the patients' ability to develop coping skills to help deal with any pain and anxiety (Field and Adams, 2001).

Pain assessment tools

Individual pain cannot be experienced by others. It is entirely subjective and will vary according to a person's physical and mental state of health, cultural expectations, degree of fatigue and previous experience of pain. Assessment of pain can be a difficult process, as practitioners have in the past had to rely almost exclusively on the patient's verbal account of it. People with a reduced capacity to express themselves through language, for example, children were at a disadvantage in receiving adequate help in obtaining pain relief.

Problems in appreciating pain experience have led to the development of pain assessment tools that use ways, other than descriptive methods to get the information across. Some tools use a scale design. For example, patients are asked to say what their pain is on a scale of one to ten, where zero is no pain and ten is the worse pain they can imagine. Other tools use pictorial depictions of different facial expressions, from happy to sad to help gauge levels of pain. In addition to degree, practitioners also need to obtain other information about a patient's pain, such as when it occurs, what exacerbates it, what relieves it, any analgesia used and how effective it is.

Pain is a common problem for tissue viability practitioners to deal with. Whereas a wound may be fairly comfortable for most of the time and pain controlled easily with regular over-the-counter preparations, dressing changes may initiate a transient period of intense pain. On these occasions a very much stronger, ideally short-acting, analgesic will be required. Alternatively, a patient with a leg ulcer may have several different pain pathologies. There may be the pain relating to the wound itself, there may be ischaemic pain in the whole leg due to a reduced arterial supply, and there may be neurological disaesthesic pain in the foot due to longstanding concomitant diabetes. Complex pain aetiologies will require a number of pain reducing treatments and strategies. It is essential to take a careful pain history, as this will ensure a more appropriate and effective use of analgesics.

Treating pain

As with every other aspect of patient care, a holistic approach is important when planning interventions to relieve pain. Analgesics are only a part, albeit a very important one, of the whole picture. Care practitioners should be also looking at ways to help reduce anxiety, improve nutrition, activity and general well-being, which will reduce the amount of analgesia required to achieve freedom from pain.

The general principle of analgesic therapy is that treatment begins with the simplest and safest preparations. If adequate pain relief is not achieved or maintained then more complex preparations are added or tried in a structured way, until analgesia is achieved. This concept of a progressive stepping up in treatment is known as an 'Analgesic Ladder' and was first produced as a guideline by the World Health Organisation (WHO) in the late 1980s (Jajad and Browman, 1995). Originally developed for the management of cancer pain, its simple premise of effectively using a range of relatively inexpensive preparations to meet the individual needs of each patient has been widely adapted for more general uses (Lawler, 2001). The version shown (*Figure 3.1*) is the adaptation of the ladder developed specifically for use with patients with painful leg ulcers attending the Leg Ulcer Clinic at Moseley Hall Hospital in Birmingham. It is tailored specifically to meet the needs of the target group who are likely to be elderly and possibly living alone. Older people can have increased susceptibility to many commonly used medicines so particular care in prescribing analgesia must be exercised (*British National Formulary* [*BNF*], 2003).

Analgesia and dressing change

Wound dressings are one of a number of nursing or medical procedures that can cause intense pain of short duration. Another example is the manipulation of a fracture prior to plastering. This type of pain, known as 'procedural' (Williams, 2003) or 'incident' pain (Lawler, 2001), is outside the scope of the 'Analgesic ladder' and requires an alternative analgesic strategy.

Changing a dressing on a patient who begins to experience pain can also be traumatic for the practitioner however gentle they are. Fear of hurting the patient could also compromise performance, as concentration is required for the multiple activities of supporting the patient, reassessing the wound and performing the skill as proficiently as possible. Any additional pressure to go quicker or to take short cuts to avoid causing pain can lead to poor practice. It is therefore in the best interests of both patient and professional that analgesia is adequate and the possible need for it anticipated. A relaxed and comfortable patient allows the practitioner to concentrate fully on the task in hand.

Complete pain relief is often difficult to achieve, as standard management for background pain is inadequate for procedural pain (Williams, 2003). What is required is a quick-acting preparation, that has a strong analgesic action but is very short lived. Patients attending out-patient clinics will have to travel home again afterwards, therefore side-effects, such as light headedness or drowsiness are highly undesirable.

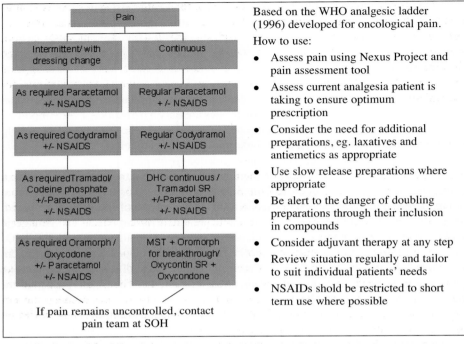

Based on the WHO analgesic ladder (1996) developed for oncological pain.

How to use:

- Assess pain using Nexus Project and pain assessment tool
- Assess current analgesia patient is taking to ensure optimum prescription
- Consider the need for additional preparations, eg. laxatives and antiemetics as appropriate
- Use slow release preparations where appropriate
- Be alert to the danger of doubling preparations through their inclusion in compounds
- Consider adjuvant therapy at any step
- Review situation regularly and tailor to suit individual patients' needs
- NSAIDs shold be restricted to short term use where possible

Figure 3.1: Moseley Hall Hospital Leg Ulcer Clinic, produced with Dr Liam Blaney

Entonox®

One of the most effective short-acting analgesics, with only minor side effects is Entonox® (Street, 2000). Entonox is a colourless and odourless compressed gas, a 50% mixture of oxygen and nitrous oxide. Introduced in 1965 (Day and Fielding, 2001), it is used widely both in hospital and in the community. Contraindications to its use are few, it being generally safe and easy to use. Self-administered by the patient, onset of analgesia is very rapid, occurring after just three or four breaths. Duration is equally short with the effects beginning to wear off immediately after inhalation ceases. Dependent on local policy, Entonox® may be used by healthcare professionals without a written prescription from a doctor (Marsden Manual of Clinical Nursing procedures, 2000). Because of its almost instantaneous effect, Entonox® is extremely useful to tissue viability practitioners, especially on those occasions where dressings are more painful than anticipated.

Helping the patient deal with pain

The tissue viability practitioner can do a great deal to help the patient cope with pain. Anxiety and fear of pain may be far worse than the pain itself. During dressing change, the practitioner should work to reduce anxiety by giving full control to the patient to halt and continue the dressing as they request. Allowing the patient to control the situation requires confidence and patience on the part of the practitioner, but fosters a relationship based on trust which, in itself, can be therapeutic.

Patients often complain that nurses don't take time sufficient to remove dressings carefully. If dressings stick ensure that they are soaked with saline or tap water, as appropriate, so that they can be removed with minimal trauma. Talking to the patient and taking an interest in their family and hobbies can also relax them and provide some distraction during a less pleasant experience. If the practitioner is also kind, appears knowledgeable and has empathy, this too can significantly improve the experience for the patient.

Aims of wound management products

There is a wide range of dressings on the market and choosing a suitable one can be a daunting task for the novice. Indeed the *British National Formulary* (*BNF*) devotes a whole appendix to them. Wound management is big business, with companies constantly expanding their ranges. For the inexperienced practitioner it can be a great source of stress and anxiety.

It is essential that all wounds are thoroughly assessed and management needs to be established prior to dressing selection. This selection is based around which product will best meet those needs and achieve the desired outcome. The practitioner requires knowledge not only of what the healing wound needs, but also of what products can do. We have touched earlier on requirements for wound healing. These are now reviewed again in the context of the properties dressings have.

Turner (1983) identified seven characteristics of an 'ideal dressing'. These are:

- maintain a moist environment
- remove excess exudate, cell debris and toxic components
- allow gaseous exchange
- be impermeable to bacteria
- provide thermal insulation to the wound surface
- be free from particulate or wound contaminants
- allow removal without trauma when changed.

Maintaining a moist environment and removing extraneous material from a wound has already been discussed. Allowing gaseous exchange is a new concept. Some dressings are more occlusive than others. Ideally, a dressing should be occlusive enough to provide a physical barrier that reduces the risk of re-injury, prevents the penetration of bacteria and maintains a moist wound environment and yet remains vapour permeable (Chang *et al*, 1998).

To Turner's original list, Morgan (2000) has added:

- safe to use
- acceptable to the patient
- cost effective
- non-flammable
- available in a range of forms and sizes.

For a dressing to be cost effective the practitioner needs to consider not only the unit price of the dressing but also the wear time and what, if any, secondary dressings may be required, which could push up the price of each individual treatments. Availability of different shapes and sizes may also make one product more cost effective than another. In selecting and using products we are using public money: if there is no difference in efficacy or acceptance by the patient we are obligated to choose the cheaper product.

Wear times

An area of anxiety for less experienced practitioners is the frequency of dressing change. If a wound is infected it will require more frequent observation to ensure adequate antibacterial therapy has been prescribed. In healthy wounds, as long as the wound remains moist, the dressing is adequately handling the exudate, there is no strike through and the dressing remains comfortable for the patient, then there is no immediate urgency to change the dressing. Changing a dressing will invariably cool the wound down, risks further minor trauma and will inevitably disrupt the wounds micro-climate. Aim to change a dressing as infrequently as possible up to a maximum of seven days.

If wounds are in a process of rapid healing or even deterioration, the point of changing the dressing is to reassess, in order to ensure that the wounds changing needs are being met. As part of becoming more familiar with products, always read the literature for advice on wear times as there may be other, for example, biochemical reasons (such as the deodorising property of a charcoal dressing becoming inactivated when the dressing is wet) for changing a dressing more frequently.

Practitioners managing venous leg ulceration with compression bandaging aim to maintain the bandages intact for seven days if the condition of the wound permits. This is because the positive effects of compression are interrupted when the bandages are replaced. It would be nonsensical to use a dressing that requires more frequent changes if this could be avoided.

Older patients may also require education on the principle of maximising wear time. This is because former practice involved daily or even more frequent dressing changes. Patients may believe that they are being neglected and need to understand why practice has changed.

The reality of the 'ideal dressing'

Of course, the 'ideal dressing' does not exist — it is merely a concept. There is no single dressing that is suitable for all wound types and through all stages of healing. Some products meet one set of criteria, others meet another set. The next section looks at the properties of dressings according to their generic grouping.

There are four main dressing groupings. They are:

- alginates
- foams
- hydrocolloids
- hydrogels.

In addition, there is a set of products that meet certain specific needs and are often used in conjunction with other products. They stand alone because in concentrating on one aspect they may meet one of the functions of the 'ideal' dressing, but fail to meet any of the others. They are:

- antibacterials
- films
- non-adherents
- deodorisers.

Alginates

Alginates are derived from seaweed and are highly absorbent. They are available as flat dressings or in rope form for use in cavities. They act via an ion exchange mechanism, absorbing serous fluid or wound exudate to become a hydrophilic gel, although different preparations have different gelling properties, and may take up to twenty-four hours to form. Those that are rich in mannuronic acid form softer, more flexible gels. Those that are rich in guluronic acid form firmer gels. This gel forming property allows the dressing to conform well to cavity wounds. Most alginates also have haemostatic properties, although some are better for this than others. For this reason, they are often used in newly created surgical wounds (Morgan, 2000). Alginates are not suitable for dry wounds and should only be used as a primary (in direct contact with the wound) dressing. If they do adhere they should be moistened with saline to allow the dressing to be removed more easily.

~ Examples are: Sorbsan® (Maersk), Kaltostat® (ConvaTec), Seasorb® (Coloplast).

Hydrofibres

Although not made of alginate and chemically more akin to hydrocolloids, hydrofibres are usually included within the alginate group because of their similarity in appearance and performance. They are up to 50% more absorbent than alginates (Morgan, 1997) and maintain their structure when wet. They are useful for packing wounds as their high tensile strength ensures that the dressing does not disintegrate on removal. Hydrofibres are also thought to have a bacteriostatic action by trapping and holding bacteria within the dressing matrix, making them useful in managing infected wounds. Use as a primary dressing only.

~ An example is: Aquacel® (ConvaTec).

Foams

These dressings are made of hydrophilic polyurethane or other compounds. They are available in a flat, shaped or cavity form. A liquid mix is also available which allows a customised wound stent to be created as the foam sets after the mixture has been poured into the wound. This preparation requires considerable skill, combined with speed, to create the dressing before the foam has solidified and, therefore, should be reserved for specific wounds.

Foams are absorbent and cope with light to medium levels of exudate and are, when used as a primary dressing, unsuitable for dry, necrotic or sloughy wounds. They are most suitable for maintaining an existing moist environment, eg. on granulating wounds. In many preparations, excess fluid is vapoured off through the outer, hydroabsorptive layer. Foams can also be used as a secondary dressing over other preparations, such as hydrogels, to maintain a moist environment. Because they can be used as the outermost dressing, they often are available with an adhesive border, which can improve their cost-effectiveness.

> ~ Examples are: Allevyn® (Smith &Nephew), Lyofoam® (SSL),
> Cavi-Care® (Smith & Nephew).

Hydrocolloids

Hydrocolloids come as flat dressings. They are either thick, which extends wear time or thin, which improves conformability. They are also available as an amorphous paste. They are more occlusive than most dressings and are used to conserve moisture, creating an environment conducive to rapid debridement which is useful for degrading necrosis and slough. Because of their occlusive properties, they should be used with caution on infected wounds. In the presence of exudate, hydrocolloids liquefy and form a gel. They are most useful for light to medium exuding wounds and can be used as a primary or secondary dressing.

Because they are applied over both the wound and the intact surrounding skin, to which they adhere, particular care must be taken in their removal to avoid skin damage. If maceration becomes a problem then friable skin may be protected by using a liquid barrier film. Hydrocolloids are also very versatile as they come in a whole range of shapes and sizes. Many can be cut to fit awkward shapes or to produce templates used to create an artificial cavity or to protect the skin from the side-effects of other therapies, eg. maggots. Others are bordered to improve adhesion or backed with foam to increase wear times.

> ~ Examples are: Granuflex® (ConvaTec), Comfeel® (Coloplast),
> DuoDERM® (ConvaTec).

Hydrogels

These are most commonly used in an amorphous form but are also available as sheet dressings. They have a high water content and although they can absorb a small amount of exudate they are mainly used to rehydrate dry wounds; indeed, they are the main products for this. Rehydrating a dry wound promotes autolysis. In an amorphous gel form they are versatile dressings as they can be used on and in wounds of all shapes and sizes. Hydogels come in tubes or pods and the required amount can be squeezed directly into the wound. If the wound is very dry, more gel will be required to rehydrate the eschar than if the wound is already moist. Avoid contact with surrounding healthy skin as maceration can occur. Most preparations are primary dressings so will generally need a secondary dressing to hold the gel in place, such as a foam or a hydrocolloid.

> ~ Examples are: Aquaform® (Maersk), Intrasite® (Smith & Nephew),
> Hydrosorb® (Hartmann).

Pared down to essentials, these four main groups will serve the needs of the majority of wounds with a few exceptions. Add four more additional dressing groups to the armoury and virtually all needs will be covered.

Antibacterials

Although they have always been included as dressings, many antibacterials should be regarded more as treatments rather than true dressings. This is because many of them meet few, if any, of the 'ideal dressing criteria' and are not designed to do so. The antibacterial preparation usually consists of a carrier, eg. an emulsive cream or sheet dressing containing an active bacteriostatic/bacteriocidal agent such as silver or iodine. This type of preparation is designed exclusively to address the bacterial milieu of a wound and no other wound care requirement. This type of product must be used in conjunction with standard wound care products.

More recently, however, dressings are being developed which combine an active agent within a modern dressing format. This ensures that the wound's general needs can be met whilst the imperative to reduce the bacterial burden is addressed. Used correctly and appropriately, these dressings could prove to be highly cost effective. Iodine, for example, is available as a hydrophyllic paste, powder or ointment.

Antibacterials are only indicated when infection is present or strongly suspected and should not be used prophylactically. Ideally, the problem organism within the wound should have been identified prior to using a product so that a dressing containing the appropriate antibacterial agent can be selected. Always read the product literature carefully for contra indications and cautions as certain products are toxic to persons with certain conditions or sensitivities and may, in any event, only be used for a limited period. Practitioners should be aware that some products may stain the tissues significantly which can mar the accuracy of some aspects of wound assessment.

Other products, such as honey and the hydrofibres, have a bacteriostatic rather than bacteriocidal action and should also be considered in the management of infected wounds (see relevant sections).

~ Examples are: Flamazine® (Smith & Nephew), Iodasorb ointment® (Smith & Nephew), Actisorb Silver 220® (Johnson & Johnson), Aquacel AG® (ConvaTec).

Films

Films have virtually no ability to handle exudate and can only be used as a primary dressing on partial-thickness or very low exuding wounds. They are, however, highly conformable and vapour permeable and are often used as secondary dressings. They are also transparent, permitting visualisation of the wound without the need to remove the dressing.

Films can be difficult to apply because their thinness and adhesiveness and require a decisive hand. Most have removable firm backings to aid application and because they stick well they can cause trauma if not removed carefully. There is a knack to this, which involves stretching the dressing away from the wound rather than simply pulling it off.

~ Examples are: Tegaderm® (3M), Opsite® (Smith & Nephew), Mefilm® (Mölnlycke).

Non-adherents

That a dressing should not cause trauma to a wound is a highly desirable quality for a primary dressing and some dressings are more successful at achieving this than others. To reduce the chances of adherence, especially where wounds are friable and would bleed easily or where pain is a particular problem, an additional non-adherent layer is sometimes used before other dressings are applied.

Non-adherent dressings are produced primarily as thin, flat, inert layers of open weave tulle or net, made of cotton or synthetic fibres which are coated with silicone or hydrocolloid or made entirely of them. This type of dressing is designed to permit interaction between the wound and the dressing of choice, while reducing the potential for adhesion. Another style of 'non-adherent' dressing, which is more truly 'low adherent' in action, consists of a polyester film over a viscose pad, which collects exudate.

The cost of these dressings varies enormously from a few pence for the polyester fibre dressings to several pounds for the silicone dressings, but their performance can also vary considerably too. Some of the silicone dressings can be worn in excess of seven days which can greatly improve their cost effectiveness (Morgan, 2000)

~ Examples are: NA Ultra® (Johnson & Johnson), Mepital® (Mölnlycke),
Urgotul® (Parema), Melolin® (Smith & Nephew)

Deodorisers

The ability to control odour is not given as one of the 'ideal' criteria for a wound dressing, but many patients are more concerned about the problem of wound odour than they are about healing rate. All wounds give off some odour and the presence of odour *per se* may have nothing to do with infection.

Some dressings, eg. hydrocolloids, give off a distinct, yet normal odour when removed. Autolysing necrotic wounds give off the strong, sweet, smell of decaying tissue and certain bacteria, eg. *pseudomonas*.

As wounds heal and begin to granulate and epithelialise, wound odour generally decreases. Malignant wounds, which do not heal, can be a particular problem because of the longstanding colonising bacteria present.

Dressings that have deodorising properties can be extremely useful in improving the patients' sense of well-being, adding greatly to their quality of life.

Charcoal is the basic constituent for most deodorising dressings and as with the non-adherent group, most of these preparations are designed to do little more than to control odour. Others in this category are primarily antibacterial products that additionally happen to control odour. Furthermore, some products are ineffective or less effective when wet. A clear understanding of the needs of the wound and the properties of each product is of particular importance to select the most cost-effective product. As with antibacterials, combined products are now becoming available that address the general needs of a wound but control odour at the same time. Depending on the preparation they can be used as primary and/or secondary dressings.

~ Examples are: Clinisorb® (CliniMed), Carbopad® (Vernon-Carus), Actisorb Silver 220® (Johnson & Johnson), CarboFLEX® (ConvaTec), Lyofoam 'C'® (SSL).

Topical antibiotics

Due to the risk of inducing antibiotic resistance, topical preparations containing antibiotics should be avoided where possible. If clinical infection is present within a wound, systemic antibiotics should be prescribed.

Topical metronidazole is, however, particularly effective in dealing with anaerobic bacteria which characteristically colonise malignant wounds, causing a lingering, pungent odour. Some preparations of metronidazole gel have been licensed for use in this particular area.

Mupericin is often prescribed for short-term use on wounds where methicillin resistant *Staphylococcus aureus* (MRSA) is present, often requiring application of two to three times per day. It is arguable whether this form of treatment is the best method or not of dealing with the problem. Disturbing the wound too frequently will slow down rather than promote healing and the MRSA will anyway be eradicated when the wound has healed.

Practical advice on the application of dressings

Wounds come in all shapes, sizes and sites. Some are considerably easier to manage than others. The nice tidy wound, usually found conveniently on the back of the forearm, that appears in promotional literature for dressings, is a far cry from the reality experienced by tissue viability practitioners every day.

This section is intended to provide a few practical solutions to some of the problems encountered in dressing wounds and covers such aspects as getting dressings to stick, applying dressings to awkward areas and dealing with excess exudate.

The first tip may be obvious, but seldom observed. Read the product information that comes with the dressings first. Many of these will have useful suggestions as to how best to apply them. For example, from reading product literature one might learn that hydrocolloids should be warmed between the palms of the hand prior to use. Warming the dressing makes it more malleable and increases its adhesive capability.

In order to be effective a dressing has to stay in place. If the dressing itself has an adhesive border or has inherent adhesive properties, as in the case of hydrocolloids, it is essential to ensure that a good seal is achieved between the skin and the dressing. There should be uninterrupted contact around the entire border of the dressing. Gaps often manifest themselves shortly after application because the skin may have been moist due to exudate or creams or the dressing has been stretched over, rather than eased around skin contours.

A particularly difficult area for less experienced practitioners to dress is the sacral area. This is because the skin fold of the natal cleft, between the buttocks and close to the anal margin, is a naturally moist area. A sacral dressing poses both moisture and contour problems. Failure to seal this area properly allows any exudate or hydrogel (if used) to come into contact with intact skin and permits any faecal soiling to get in under the dressing.

Prepare the surrounding area well. Clean the area around the wound and ensure it is dry and free from greasy preparations. Avoid overspill of hydrogels or other products used on the wound, onto the intact skin. If the skin still feels damp, a hair dryer (on the cool setting) will dry the skin more thoroughly and less traumatically than further rubbing with towels or gauze. Start with the natal cleft first. Having an assistant to gently separate the buttocks to create a flatter surface is a real boon. If a square or rectangular dressing has to be used, often it may be easier to apply the dressing diagonally, with one of the corners dipping into the natal cleft. Above all, do not stretch the dressing edge to get it to fit, but mould it gently into place without any tension. Once that part is secure, work along the margins, using a rolling motion, until the dressing is in place. Hampton (1996) suggests placing the hand over the dressing for a few minutes to ensure a good seal. If the skin of the natal cleft is particularly moist through sweat, the use of a prescribed anti-perspirant, such as aluminium chloride, might be useful.

If the area around any wound is friable or excoriated, a barrier film, such as Cavilon may be useful. This type of product should be alcohol free, sterile and safe to use on broken areas. This film coats the damaged skin and provides a dry base for the dressing to adhere to. It also protects the skin from further maceration.

If wounds are to be covered with bandages anyway, as in the case of leg ulcers, it is often not necessary to use adhesive tape to secure dressings directly onto potentially friable skin. Tubular cotton bandage is ideal in this instance for holding dressings in place (*Figures 3.2* and *3.3*), especially if there is a lot of them. Start by cutting a length of the tubular cotton slightly longer than the lower leg. Have all the dressings ready, but start by putting the tubular cotton over the foot first. Then dress the leg in sections, as required, rolling the tubular bandage into place as you move up the leg. An extra pair of hands is useful here! Any slippage while other dressings are positioned, can be easily corrected later, before the first strip bandage is applied. The excess of the tubular bandage can be folded over and secured to the strip bandage layer with tape or more bandaging, if to be used. Small tubular bandages are also particularly useful for helping to secure dressings on fingers and toes and larger ones for stump dressings.

Product information often contains diagrams of how to cut particular shapes to cover contoured areas, but if you are intending to cut a dressing, check that the dressing is suitable for cutting first. The integrity of some dressings may be destroyed by cutting them. Ropes and cavity fillers are usually used for deeper wounds, but by using a circular cutting technique, a flat hydrofibre dressing can be cut into one long strip and used as packing (Dunford, 1997).

When necrotic wounds on convex areas such as the heels require the use of hydrogel to debride, there is the danger that when the secondary dressing is applied the gel will be pushed on to the healthy skin. To avoid this, a template of hydrocolloid can be made (*Figures 3.4* and *3.5*). Take a flat dressing and cut a hole into it the same size as the wound. Secure the template in place leaving the wound exposed. The thickness of the hydrocolloid has now created a small cavity, into which the gel can be applied, and then cover with a secondary dressing that will maintain the moist environment.

Wound exudate is often difficult to manage. Whilst other management strategies are being employed to control the situation, such as systemic antibiotics for infection or elevation and compression for venous leg ulcers, where exudate is excessive the practitioner may be faced with a wound that becomes sodden within a few hours. Even the most absorbent dressing has a limit. The use of barrier films to protect the skin surrounding the wound is essential. Other strategies can include using a flexible, open weave, non-adherent silicone dressing next to the wound and replacing the outer dressing only, as they become wet. Where sinuses are constantly leaking the continence advisor may have a solution. Stoma bags, especially those with granules that form a gel in the presence of liquid may be particularly useful. Vacuum-assisted closure is an excellent means of controlling exudate providing the wound is suitable.

If wounds are particularly challenging, because they are excessively wet or malodorous or are fungating or in intimate areas, a particularly sensitive approach is required. Patients need to know that the practitioner is not shocked or overwhelmed by the problems however considerable they are. If you meet with a difficult problem, do seek help. In the field of tissue viability, some new challenge is sure to crop up from time to time! Make use of other colleagues, including the multidisciplinary team. You may not have encountered that particular problem before but it is likely that someone else has and will be glad to help. Often the solution comes through adapting something used in one area, for use in another. The use of stoma bags for exuding sinuses is an example.

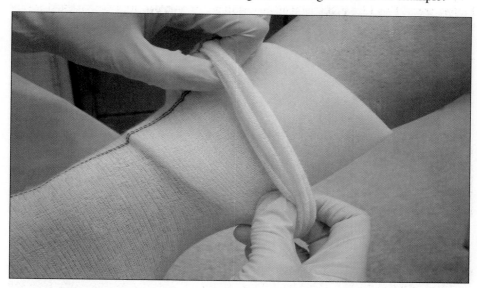

Figure 3.2: Bandage application — 1

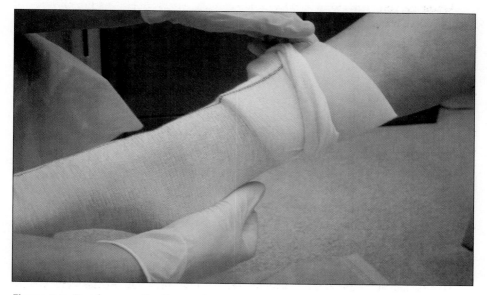

Figure 3.3: Bandage application — 2

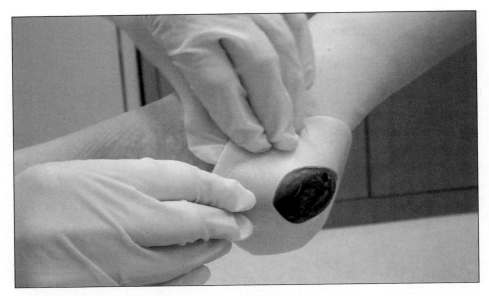

Figure 3.4: Hydrocolloid template – 1

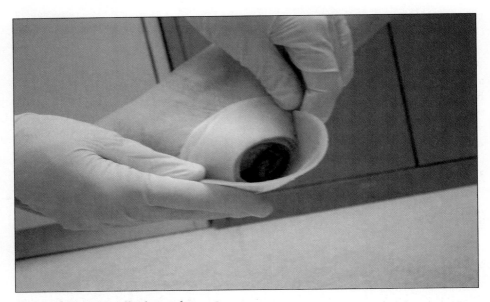

Figure 3.5: Hydrocolloid template – 2

Wound treatment matrix

There are many guides to help practitioners select suitable dressings. An example of such a 'wound treatment matrix' matrix is shown in *Appendix 2*.

Cost-effectiveness

As suggested, the combining of dressing types to create a third hybrid may result in a product that will be cheaper to use overall, possibly less bulky and perhaps more effective. However, there are times when combined products can be more expensive because they meet the needs of only a small group of patients and quantity saving cannot be made. In addition, some products are not that well designed, and the properties of the various components may actually counteract one another.

Formularies used in hospitals are likely to contain a more restricted range of dressings than is available on prescription. Dressings form a large part of the pharmacy budget and by buying in bulk, one type of foam or one type of alginate, cost reductions can be negotiated. Hospital-based practitioners should seek advice from their pharmacy departments when considering using non-formulary products. In the community, actual prices are given in the *British National Formulary* (*BNF*).

In addition to the cost of dressings, practitioners need also to consider the cost of other wound care items, eg. adhesive tape. An island dressing might turn out to be a cheaper option than one fixed in position with gauze and tape. Wear times can also affect costs considerably: products with a higher unit price but longer wear time may represent better value for money than the reverse.

Government advice on selection of wound management products

With the advent of nurse prescribing the National Prescribing Centre (NPC) (http://www.npc.co.uk) produced a series of pages and bulletins designed to help nurses select wound management products wisely. This has been helpful to practitioners, who having successfully negotiated the choice of generic group, still found the last hurdle of selecting the actual brand very confusing.

The advice from the NPC is unambiguous. It states that although there is evidence that modern wound dressing products do have a role in wound healing, no single product is suitable for use in all wounds and at all stages of healing. Choice of dressing should be based on using the cheapest effective dressing, acceptable to both patient and prescriber, which is suitable for the stage of healing of the wound. Knowledge of the actual unit cost of products *per se* and in relation to sizes available is essential if nurses are to follow that advice responsibly.

Patient concordance

Practitioners should always regard the patient as a partner in decisions regarding the management of their wound. In order for the patient to perform this role adequately and to be able to make informed choices, sufficient time should be allocated for patient education. Patients need to know the basics of wound healing and the rationale for dressing selection. We used to speak of patient compliance, whereby patients complied with treatments decided for them by others. Now we speak more of concordance, which suggests a more equal relationship.

Although achieving concordance places the onus on the practitioner to inform and involve the patient in his or her care, it also places a hitherto under utilised responsibility on the patient to 'own' their wound. For some patients this idea may be difficult to accept and may cause anxiety. They may initially prefer the practitioner to assume and maintain full responsibility. Considerable tact and patience is required in helping the patient to develop their knowledge and skills and thereby gain the confidence to vocalise their wishes.

Reflective activity

Consider a wound you have assessed and dressed recently. Could you have used other strategies or products that could have improved the outcome for the patient? Could you also have done this and achieved cost savings too?

Patient scenario three

Look again at Mr Skelton's pressure ulcer, which is shown in *Figure 2.7 (p. 21)*. Complete a wound treatment plan (either one from your clinical practice area or by using the one shown in the appendices). Include all relevant aspects including aims of treatment, wound cleansing, dressing selection, skin care, pain management and any thing else that you consider relevant to his care.

Key points

❖ Good wound and patient assessment provides the basis for selecting the most appropriate wound healing therapy.

❖ If using a new product or one you haven't used for a long time always read the product literature and *BNF* to familiarise yourself with product indications and contra-indications, what the product is and isn't licensed for, sizes, shapes and preparations available and relative product costs.

❖ Be wary of claims made by product manufacturers who are keen to sell their products. If, in doubt, get your advice from government publications or websites or other independent sources.

❖ Products are constantly being withdrawn and added to making it very difficult to keep fully up-to-date. Therefore, concentrate initially on getting a grasp of the 4 + 4 main dressing types, gradually widening your knowledge of the product range of each dressing type as you gain confidence.

References

Brennan SS (1985) The effect of antiseptics on the healing wound: a study using the rabbit ear. *Chamber British Journal of Surgery* **72**: 780–82

Briggs M, Torra I Bou (2003) Pain at wound dressing changes: a guide to management. In: Pain at wound dressing changes. European Wound Management Association, Position Statement. Medical Education Partnership Ltd, London

British National Formulary (2003) British Medical Association & Royal Pharmaceutical Society of Great Britain, Pharmaceutical Press, Oxford

Chang YC, Cho MD, Lo JS (1998) Dressing the part. *Dermatologic Clinics* **16**(1): 25–47

Collier M (2003) Wound bed preparation: theory to practice. *Nurs Standard* **17**(36): 45–55

Cooper R, Lawrence JC (1996) Micro-organisms and wounds. *J Wound Care* **5**(5): 233–6

Day A, Fielding C (2001) Using entonox in the community. *J Wound Care* **10**(4): 108

Dowsett C (2002) The role of the nurse in wound bed preparation. *Nurs Standard* **16**(44): 69–76

Dunford C (1997) A guide to management of cavity wounds. *Nurs Times Know How*: 6 August

Ennis W, Meneses P (2000) Wound healing at the local level: the stunned wound. *Ostomy Wound Management* **46**(1): 39–48

Griffiths RD, Fernandez RS, Ussia CA (2001) Is tap water a safe alternative to normal saline for wound irrigation in the community setting? *J Wound Care* **10**(10): 407–11

Hampton S (1996) Dressing awkward areas. *Nurs Times Know How*: 25 September

Jajad AR, Browman GP (1995) The WHO analgesic ladder for cancer pain and management. *JAMA* **274**(23): 1870–73

Lawler K (2001) Factfile analgesia. *Prof Nurse* **17**(4): 219–20

Lawrence JC (1996) The use of antiseptics in wound care. *J Wound Care* **5**(1): 44–7

Lock PM (1980) The effects of temperature and mitotic activity at the edge of experimental wounds. In: Sundell B, ed. Symposium on Wound Healing: Plastic Surgery and Dermatology Annab Molindal, Lindgrey A and Soner B, Switzerland

Mallett J, Dougherty L (2000) *The Royal Marsden Hospital Manual of Clinical Nursing Procedures*. 5th edn. Blackwell Science, Oxford

Mertz PM, Ovington LG (1993) Wound healing microbiology. *Dermatalogic Clinics* **11**(4): 739–47

Moffatt C, Franks PJ, Hollinsworth H (2003) Understanding wound pain and trauma: an international perspective. In: Pain at wound dressing changes. European Wound Management Association, Position Statement. Medical Education Partnership Ltd, London

Morgan DA (2000) *Formulary of Wound Management Products*. 8th edn (revised). Euromed Publications, Surrey, UK

Oliver L (1997) Wound cleansing. *Nurs Standard* **11**(20): 47–56

Schultz GS, Sibbald RG, Falanga V, Ayello EA, Dowsett C, Harding K *et al* (2003) Wound bed preparation: a systematic approach to wound management. *Wound Rep Regen* **11**(2): 1–28

Street D (2000) A practical guide to giving entonox. *Nurs Times* **96**(34): 47–8

Mallett J, Dougherty L, eds (2000) *The Royal Marsden Hospital Manual of Clinical Nursing Procedures*. 5th edn. Blackwell Science, Oxford

Turner TD (1983) Absorbents and Wound Dressings April Supplement to Nursing the Add on J Clinical Nursing 1-7

Winter GD (1962) Formation of the scab and the rate of epithelialisation of superficial wounds in the skin of the young domestic pig. *Nature* 193: 293–4

Williams H (2003) This fast acting analgesia is not just for maternity and A&E. *Nurs Times* **99**(5): 33

Wood RAB (1976) Disintegration of cellulose dressings in open granulating wounds. *Br Med J* **785**: 1444–45

Wound Care Formulary (2002) South Birmingham Primary Care NHS Trust

Chapter 4

Specific wound types

This chapter looks at a number of wound types that you will encounter during your professional practice. It will provide you with a general understanding of aetiology and awareness of current assessment and management principles.

Surgical wounds

Definition

Surgical wounds are formed from incisions that are usually undertaken in a sterile environment. There are a number of methods of closing surgical wounds (*Table 4.1*). However, the majority are closed using sutures and heal by primary intention. Surgical wounds should be closed with good opposition and without undue tension on the skin edges and need to be supported with adequate post-operative care (Leaper and Gottrup, 1998). There were over six million operations undertaken in the NHS in England and Wales in 1998/1999 (National Institute for Clinical Excellence [NICE], 2001). With the changes in health care provision and the use of day surgery facilities an increasing number of these patients will be discharged home very rapidly following surgery.

Table 4.1: Methods of surgical wound closure		
Description	**Type of surgery**	**Implications**
Primary wound closure	Incisional surgery, skin edges brought together with good opposition • sutures (deep tension for • staples/clips (skin layers) • surgical glue (facial lacerations)	Usually clean wounds. Skin closure will occur within 6–12 hours. By 48 hours the tissue will be sufficiently knitted together to prevent bacterial invasion
Delayed primary closure (early closure)	Skin closure delayed for a few days (usually within 8 days)	Usually undertaken when there is a risk of infection, such as abscess or from trauma
Secondary closure (late closure)	Skin closure delayed for a longer period (10–14 days), granulation tissue may be present	Wound may be dirty or contaminated and is left until it is clean and free from infection before suturing
Secondary intention healing	Wound not closed but left to heal by granulation	Appropriate moist wound healing agents will be required to promote healing and to prevent pain on removal

The main priorities following surgery are to promote healing, prevent infection and to restore normal function as early as possible. The majority of sutured wounds heal without complication as this is related to the overall health of the patient and the skill of the surgeon. The NICE guidance document on difficult to heal surgical wounds, states that there are no reliable figures for the number of difficult to heal surgical wounds within the NHS but that estimates of 21,000 have been given. Even if this figure is an under estimation, it still represents a small percentage of the surgical wounds overall.

Pre-operative considerations

It is important to undertake a holistic assessment of surgical patients pre-operatively to establish any potential barriers to wound healing (Watret and White, 2001). If any potential problems are identified then efforts should be made to rectify them prior to surgery.

Partridge (1998) suggests that the following should be included in this assessment:

- Nutritional state: good nutritional status results in fewer postoperative complications, better wound healing and a speedier recovery. Obese patients are more prone to wound breakdown.
- Underlying disease-state: patients with diabetes are more at risk of infection and have reduced wound tensile strength. Peripheral vascular disease may also be present which will reduce blood supply. Malignant disease or other chronic medical conditions will contribute to delayed healing (NICE, 2001). Drug therapy (ie. steroids, cytotoxic drugs, radiotherapy) can also affect healing adversely.
- Age: Physiological changes related to ageing can slow the rate and quality of healing (Desai, 1997).
- Hospital stay: the length of hospital stay pre-operatively can influence the postoperative recovery rate. Hospital stay can be prolonged because of pre-existing disease or trauma.

Wound infection

Some surgical incisions become infected, which can result in considerable morbidity and increased cost to the health service. In many instances, these infections do not become obvious until after the patient is discharged (Sharp and McLaws, 2001). The chances of developing a wound infection are increased if the surgery involves body cavities in which there is necrotic, infected or dirty tissue, as contamination will occur during the surgery (Sharp and McLaws, 2001). Colorectal surgery is an example of this, particularly in emergency cases. Infection can result in wound dehiscence, in which the suture line breaks down and separates, either partially or completely (*Figure 4.1*).

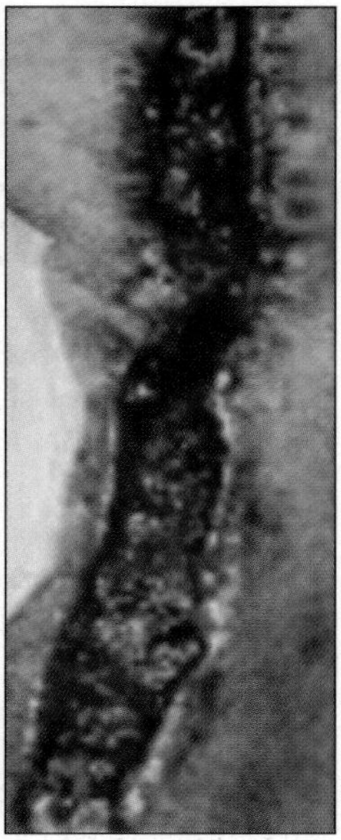

Pre-operative skin preparation is an important component of infection control. If hair removal if necessary, it should take place as near to the time of surgery as possible. The use of depilatory creams is preferable as shaving can result in skin trauma (Partridge, 1998). The skin needs to be clean prior to surgery, and showering has been shown to remove more skin micro-organisms

Figure 4.1: Wound dehiscence

43

than bathing. Baths can increase the risk of infection if they are not cleaned adequately between patients. Handwashing between patient contact is often cited as the greatest factor in preventing cross-infection (Partridge, 1998).

> ### *Reflective activity*
>
> Reflect back on situations where you were involved in the management of surgical patients. Were there any occasions when a patient developed a wound breakdown? What where the factors that lead to this, and how could the situation have been avoided? Would you change any aspect of their wound management?

Care of post-operative wounds

Post-operative wounds should be left undisturbed unless there are visible signs of infection. These may present as wound discharge, abnormal swelling and increased pain and the patient feeling unwell. Discolouration could signify haematoma formation. Wound dehiscence, in which there is a complete breakdown of the sutures, can be the consequence of infection and haematoma formation, as well as the result of poor surgical technique. It is regarded as a surgical emergency and may require immediate return to theatre for re-suturing (Robson *et al*, 1998).

As there will be adequate wound repair after forty-eight hours in the majority of patients, it has been suggested that wound dressings are not required after this time (Chrintz *et al*, 1989). Dressings do, however, prevent sutures from catching on clothing and provide a cosmetic cover (Ballard and Baxter, 2000). The use of film dressings may help to reduce incisional pain for a longer period of time (Briggs, 1996). Dressings will also be required if there is any leakage of exudate. Sutures, staples and clips need to be removed at the appropriate time. If left in place too long they may cause excess scarring and become a focus for infection, such as a stitch abscess or sinus (Harding and Jones, 1996). Wound drains are used where there is any dead space that could result in fluid collection. These will also need careful observation for signs of infection and to ensure that they maintain their vacuum. Partridge (1998), states that although there is a lack of empirical evidence, it is safer in terms of tissue trauma to release the vacuum prior to removal.

Patients often feel anxious about these removal procedures and so careful explanation and reassurance will be helpful to them. If the wound starts to gap then alternative sutures should be removed and Steri-strips used to re-oppose the edges. A strict aseptic technique must be used for any wound procedure.

Dressing selection

The majority of surgical wounds are dressed in theatre with traditional low-adherent cellulose dressings. It could be argued that as most surgical wounds heal without any problems, that these relatively cheap dressings are adequate and cost effective. They can, however, result in wound adherence as a result of dried blood products. This can cause pain, trauma and anxiety at dressing change. They are also not waterproof. If dressings are required post-operatively, the use of a non-adherent dressing that permits bathing should be considered. Examples include, thin hydrocolloids, foams, film island dressing or waterproof post-operative dressings. These may prove more appropriate and acceptable to the patient (Ballard and Baxter, 2000). It is important to apply any dressing to the skin without stretching the skin. The resultant shearing forces can cause blistering.

Wounds healing by secondary intention

Dressing selection is an important component in the care of these wounds and should be based on careful assessment of the wound and patient. Modern dressings may have a beneficial effect on outcomes, such as pain, odour and exudate management compared with traditional gauze dressings (NICE, 2001).

Traditional products, such as proflavine–impregnated gauze, are frequently used, especially in cavity wounds such as pilonidal sinus excision or abscess drainage. Unfortunately, these dressings are prone to dry out and to traumatise the wound on removal. It is not uncommon for patients to require the use of opiates, Entonox gas or even a general anaesthetic in order to cope with the pain. Foster and Moore (1997) have shown that the use of a more appropriate dressing (in this case a hydrofibre dressing), can result in significant reductions in pain. They also reported that as patients stated that they would be happy to have their first dressing change undertaken at home, this could result in considerable cost savings. It has also been suggested that this type of dressing may play a role in the reduction of infection. Their ability to bind bacteria will reduce dispersal and consequently cross-infection risk (White, 2001).

Vacuum-assisted wound closure (VAC) is now frequently used for many surgical wounds and is often applied immediately after the procedure. It is also being used for the management of wound dehiscence.

Watret and White (2001) suggest that certain criteria (*Figure 4.2*) should be considered when selecting a wound dressing for secondary healing or difficult to heal surgical wounds.

Key points

- ❖ Wound healing will depend on the health of the patient, extent of the surgery and nature of surgical closure. Surgical techniques used include primary closure, delayed primary closure, secondary closure or the use of secondary intention healing.

- ❖ Efforts should be made to rectify any potential barriers to healing such as poor nutrition and underlying disease state, prior to surgery.

- ❖ Dressing selection is an important component of post-operative care. Modern dressings may have a beneficial effect on outcomes such as pain, odour and exudate management compared with gauze dressings.

Criteria	Advantages	Examples
Conformability	Will aid patient comfort and mobility and stay in place	Alginate, foam cavity dressings hydrofibre
Cohesive	Will not fall apart on removal, particularly important for tracking wounds	Hydrofibre, some alginates
Non-adherent	Less pain and trauma on removal	Foams, hydrofibre, alginates, hydrocolloids
Absorbent	Dressings will not be prone to strike through and will not cause maceration. Longer wear time	Foams, hydrofibre, alginates, hydrocolloids
Waterproof	Able to permit showering	Hydrocolloids, films, adhesive foams
Avoid cross-infection	Prevent dispersal of bacteria on removal, may also have antibacterial properties within the dressing	Hydrofibre, hydrocolloids, silver containing dressings
Easy to use	Easy to apply and to remove. May help reduce patient anxiety at dressing change. Will also reduce waste if dressings are applied successfully each time. Patients may be able to undertake own dressings	Foams, hydrofibre, alginates, hydrocolloids, hydrogels
Available in the community	To ensure continuity of care and to maintain patient confidence	Many of the above

Figure 4.2: Criteria to be considered when selecting dressing (Watret and White, 2001)

Pressure ulceration

Definition

Pressure ulcers are areas of localised cellular damage to the skin and underlying tissues caused by pressure, shear and frictional forces. They usually occur over bony prominences such as sacrum, heels, and hips by the action of compressing the soft tissue between the support surface and the bone. The amount of damage incurred will be dependent on the magnitude, duration and direction of the loading and also the individual's response to this. They can occur in other areas of the body where skin is exposed to these damaging forces, such as from lying on catheter tubes, rolled up anti-emboli stockings or from wearing ill-fitting shoes.

Impact of pressure ulcers

Unfortunately, pressure ulcers represent an all too familiar problem to most of us and there are few areas of health care where patients will not be at some degree of risk. Pressure ulcers occur across all age groups, social class and race and have been reported in maternity (Malone, 2000) and paediatric units (Curley, 2003).

Costs

The cost of pressure ulceration is huge. They carry a high human cost as they can result in much pain, discomfort, anxiety and frustration. They can prolong the rehabilitation process and prevent the patient from returning to normal activities. In cases of extreme pressure damage, resulting infection and osteomyelitis may prove life threatening. In a recent European survey that included the UK, 18.1% of hospital patients were found to have pressure ulcers (Clark, Bours and Defloor, 2003). The true economic cost of pressure ulceration is unknown, particularly in the community, however a recent estimate of the total cost has been given as £1.4–£2.1 billion annually (4% of the total NHS expenditure). Most of this cost is nursing time (Bennett *et al*, 2004). Costs for the increasing number of litigation cases is an added expense (Tingle, 1997).

Policies and guidelines

In recent years, pressure ulcer prevention has received a lot of attention from the Government and NHS as it is seen as a key quality indicator (DoH, 1993). NHS Trusts and organisations are expected to provide guidance on how they should be prevented. The Royal College of Nursing (RCN) issued evidence-based guidelines in 2000. These were then followed by the publication of *Inherited Clinical Guidelines* produced by the NHS National Institute for Clinical Excellence (NICE) in 2001, which have recently been updated (2003). The European Pressure Ulcer Advisory Panel (EPUAP) also produced guidelines in 1998 with the aim of improving pressure ulcer prevention and management across Europe. Pressure ulcer prevention has also been included as one of the eight original benchmarks included in the *Essence of Care*, clinical practice benchmark programme (DoH, 2003).

Causes of pressure ulceration

Tissue will break down when exposed to prolonged or high levels of pressure combined with other variables such as shear, friction and moisture. It is often the combination of forces, which leads to tissue distortion and destruction. Vessels within the microcirculation, such as capillaries and lymphatics are compressed and occluded which, if prolonged, can lead to ischaemia and tissue death. It is important to be able to recognise situations where a patient is exposed to these forces.

Pressure

This is a perpendicular load of force (such as the patient's body weight) exerted on a unit of area (eg. the sacrum), and is considered to be the major force involved in pressure ulceration (Bennett and Lee, 1986). As well as causing local capillary occlusion, pressure can also be transmitted through the tissues between the skin surface and underlying bone structure, compressing all the intermediate tissue. McClemont (1984) has described the resultant pressure gradient as a 'cone of pressure'. The pressure within the deeper tissues can be three to five times greater than that experienced on the skin. This is why pressure ulcers can break down to reveal cavities, as damage has been taking place undetected within the deep tissues. Pressure exerted on the skin is measured and is referred to as 'interface pressure'.

Normal response to pressure

As a result of research by Landis on healthy volunteers (1930), the pressure within capillaries is often quoted as being 32mm Hg. It is assumed that any pressure applied to the skin greater than this will occlude capillaries. However, the capillary closing pressure for certain groups, such as the elderly may be much lower. The pressure exerted on our skin during the course of normal activities regularly exceeds the figure of 32mmHg; for example, the pressure exerted on the skin when sitting on a firm chair may be between 100–200mmHg. Fortunately, the body is designed to be able to cope with this — why is this?

Figure 4.3 illustrates how we are protected from tissue damage by our ability to feel pain and discomfort and to move so as to redistribute our load and to keep our circulation intact. This is an ongoing process and one that we rarely think of. Each person has an individual tolerance of these forces. Halfens (2000)

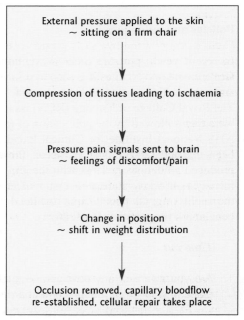

External pressure applied to the skin
~ sitting on a firm chair

↓

Compression of tissues leading to ischaemia

↓

Pressure pain signals sent to brain
~ feelings of discomfort/pain

↓

Change in position
~ shift in weight distribution

↓

Occlusion removed, capillary bloodflow re-established, cellular repair takes place

Figure 4.3: Normal response to pressure

states that the best indicators for the risk of pressure ulcers are the intensity and duration of compression and shearing forces and the tissue tolerance of pressure and oxygen deprivation.

Shear

Shearing forces result in layers of tissue moving in opposing planes. The skeleton and deep fascia slide downward with gravity while the skin and upper fascia remain in the original position. Damage is caused when underlying fibres and subcutaneous tissue are ripped and separated. Shear will enhance the effects of pressure and will result in tissue distortion; the resulting damage will occur in a shorter period of time.

Shearing usually occurs during moving and handling of patients. When a patient is sitting up in bed the normal response is to slide down. If they are then lifted up the bed incorrectly, the shearing forces will be introduced again. Simply elevating the foot end of the bed slightly, or using the knee break on a profiling bed will prevent sliding. Shearing forces can also be introduced when a patient is transferring from bed to chair. Patient and staff awareness of correct methods of moving and handling is vital to prevent the damaging effects of shearing.

Friction

Friction occurs when two surfaces rub together and is enhanced in the presence of heat and moisture. Inappropriate turning of patients where the skin is dragged across the sheets, rubbing from clothing and straps or from armrests are all examples of frictional damage.

Moisture

The skin can be exposed to moisture through incontinence, perspiration and wound drainage. Although these substances may contain factors other than moisture that irritate the skin, moisture alone can make the skin more susceptible to frictional forces (Agency for Health Care Policy and Research [AHCPR], 1994). Consider how easy it is to get foot blisters when your feet are hot and sweaty on a summer's day.

Identifying patients at risk

The most important factors in preventing pressure ulcers are to identify those who are at risk and then alleviate the forces that cause pressure damage.

There are numerous intrinsic risk factors that will increase the susceptibility to pressure damage. The *Inherited Clinical Guidelines* (NICE, 2001; 2003) lists the following risk factors:

- reduced mobility or immobility
- sensory impairment
- acute illness
- level of consciousness
- extremes of age
- vascular disease
- severe chronic or terminal illness
- previous history of pressure damage
- malnutrition and dehydration.

Pressure damage can occur rapidly in a vulnerable person; therefore, a thorough risk assessment is required as soon as possible on entry into any episode of care. The EPUAP pressure ulcer prevention guidelines suggest that this assessment should also include general medical condition, skin assessment, moisture and incontinence, nutrition and pain.

There are a variety of risk assessment tools available to help in this process. Tools commonly used within the UK include Waterlow (1985), Norton (1962) and the Braden scale (1987). These tools are used to provide a systematic evaluation of the individual's at-risk status and to provide a predictive numerical score (Culley, 2002). The advantages and disadvantages of using such tools are shown in *Table 4.2*.

Table 4.2: Advantages and disadvantages of risk assessement scoring systems

Advantages	Disadvantages
Act as an 'aide memoire'	Weak predictive values
Prompt to intervene	May not be reliable
Focuses attention on pressure ulcers	'cut-off' points for risk, ie. low, high
Provides a grade of risk for audit purposes	Usually only completed on admission when only limited information may be available or known
Assist in the documentation of risk	May not lead to skin inspection or predict individual response to pressure
Many are nationally recognised and respected	Many do not include friction, shear and moisture

Using a risk assessment tool is only helpful when it is used as part of a complete prevention programme. Simply using a risk assessment scale without knowledge, clinical skills, time and equipment to prevent pressure ulcers will not have the desired effect (Halfens, 2000). There is no evidence that risk assessment scales are better than nurses' judgement in identifying patients at risk (NHS Centre for Reviews and

Dissemination, 1995). It is also important to update any assessment on a regular basis or when there is any change in the patient's condition. Your knowledge base of a patient will obviously increase with time spent with them, it is important to update your original assessment using this additional information. There is a need to think ahead, for example, a surgical nurse will need to recognise pre-operatively the post-operative needs of a patient scheduled for major surgery on the basis of prior knowledge and experience, and provide the necessary equipment and resources (Nixon and McGough, 2001).

Patient scenario four

Identify all possible risk factor that are relevant to Mr Skelton. What level of risk do you think Mr Skelton presents with in terms of developing further pressure damage ?

Risk factors:

Level of risk:

Although risk assessment scales can be an important starting point, they are no substitute for using your clinical judgement when assessing patients. One of the most important components of this is skin inspection.

The EPUAP guidelines (1998) state that skin should be inspected and documented daily and any changes should be recorded as soon as they are observed. This skin inspection should take into account the following:

- bony prominences (sacrum, heels, hips, ankles, elbows, occiput)
- condition of the skin: dryness, cracking, erythema, maceration, fragility, heat and induration.

Clothing may need to be removed in order to undertake a thorough skin inspection which includes anti-emboli stockings. These can be a cause of skin damage (*Figure 4.4*).

Skin inspection is an important skill and the tissue viability practitioner should be aware of what is a normal and abnormal response to pressure. Reactive hyperaemia is a normal response whereas a non-blanching hyperaemia is indicative of micro-circulatory damage. The following definitions serve as a useful guide.

Hyperaemia definitions (NICE, 2003)

❖ *Reactive hyperaemia*

The characteristic bright flush of the skin associated with the increased volume of the pulse on the release of an obstruction to the circulation, or a vascular flush following the release of an occlusion of the circulation which is a direct response to incoming arterial blood.

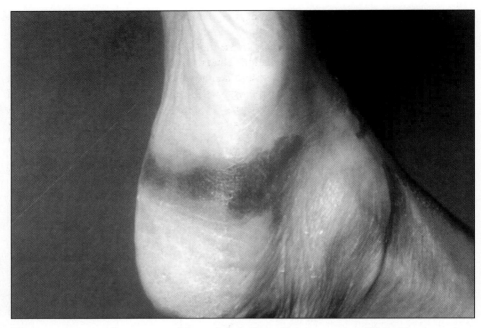

Figure 4.4: Pressure damage caused by anti-emboli stockings, courtesy of K Gerbhardt

❖ *Blanching hyperaemia*

The distinct erythema caused by reactive hyperaemia, when the skin blanches or whitens if light finger pressure is applied, indicating that the patient's microcirculation is intact.

❖ *Non-blanching hyperaemia*

Indicated when there is no skin colour change of the erythema when light finger pressure is applied, indicating a degree of microcirculatory disruption often associated with other clinical signs, such as blistering, induration and oedema.

Blisters, discoloration, localised heat, oedema and localised induration should also be observed for (NICE, 2003). Patients may also tell you that they are aware of soreness and discomfort. It is difficult to identify hyperaemia in dark skin; therefore, the following should be observed for: purplish/bluish tinge to the skin and again localised heat, oedema and discoloration.

Opportunities such as toileting, washing and moving patients can be used for skin inspection. To inspect the feet, particularly the heels, anti-emboli stockings should be removed daily. Those who are able should be encouraged, following training, to inspect their skin themselves. For wheelchair users this may involve the use of a mirror (NICE, 2001, 2003).

Whenever skin inspection reveals any potential or actual skin damage, the first course of action is to reposition the person off this area immediately.

Documenting findings

Risk assessments need to be documented and must lead onto appropriate care planning. Both the risk assessment and care plan will need regular reviews and updates. Any repositioning and mobility schedules should also be clearly documented to ensure that all staff involved with the patient complies with them. The *Code of Professional Conduct* (UKCC, 1992), states that all patients have a right to receive information about their condition and so they should be fully informed about their level of risk and what they can do to prevent any skin damage. The recent NICE guidelines (2003) state that all patients vulnerable to pressure ulcers, should be provided with both verbal and written information on all aspects of prevention. A recent professional misconduct case study (Castledine, 2003) highlights the consequences of not providing this information.

Reflective activity

Think back to any form of patient assessment that you have undertaken recently. How much information did you give to the patient and their carers/family? How could you improve upon this in the future?

Effective preventative measures

There is general consensus that the best prevention strategies involve skin care, individualised mobility programmes and appropriate use of support surfaces.

Skin care

As moisture can weaken the skin and contribute to its breakdown, any source of moisture (eg. incontinence) should be controlled. The skin should always be treated with respect and rubbing avoided. Emollients and moisturisers may be required for dry skins; barrier creams may also be required.

❖ Mobility and repositioning programmes

The aim of keeping the patient mobile is to protect against the adverse effects of pressure, shear and friction. Regular repositioning will be required if they are not able to keep mobile. The optimal frequency for repositioning patients is not known, although traditionally two-hourly changes have been advocated. In reality, patients are probably not repositioned as frequently as they should be (Clark, 1998). Because of the nursing time implications of constantly moving patients, pressure-relieving equipment is frequently used. It is important to avoid positioning vulnerable patients on their sacrum and trochanters. Positioning techniques such as the thirty-degree tilt can also be considered (Preston, 1988). This technique uses pillows to tilt the patient's sacrum off the bed at a thirty-degree angle, while also lifting the heels off the bed by using additional pillows. This position is comfortable and effective but the patient will need to be frequently checked to ensure that they have stayed in this position.

The only reliable indicator of checking whether your repositioning schedule is effective is by checking the skin for signs of marking. All efforts will be undermined if ineffective moving and handling techniques are used, as these will result in friction and shearing forces being introduced.

❖ *Sitting*

Patients are at greater risk of developing skin damage when sitting out in chairs as up to 75% of their body weight is transferred through a relatively small surface area (the buttocks). Shearing forces are also easily introduced when the patient slides down, usually resulting in them 'sacral' sitting'. The most common position that patients with seating problems adopt is that of a posterior pelvic tilt (Collins, 2001). In this position, the sacrum and coccyx take most of the person's weight. The feet are often pushed forward in an attempt to offer support which can result in heel pressure ulcers. The increased risk associated with sitting is seldom fully recognised and patients are often left to sit in chairs for long periods of time. Cushions may be used to prolong the sitting time for patients. However, these may alter the patient's position and posture (ie. feet may no longer be on the floor) and can make the situation worse. The EPUAP and NICE guidelines suggest that any person who is acutely ill and is at risk of developing pressure ulcers should avoid uninterrupted sitting out of bed and that, generally, this should not exceed two hours. A study by Gerbhardt and Bliss (1994), showed that in a control group of patients whose sitting times were limited to less than two hours, as well as a reduction in pressure ulcers, there was also a reduction in constipation, chest and urinary tract infections and immobility. Various strategies can be used to ensure mobility schedules are adhered to; these include turning clocks and charts, and ensuring that patients are aware of the need to move and have access to a clock or watch.

There will be patients who will need to spend substantial periods of time in a chair or wheelchair. It is important that they are provided with seating that is the correct height and also a pressure-relieving cushion suitable for their individual needs. Advice from 'a trained assessor' should be sought regarding correct seating positions (NICE, 2003). When a patient is being reintroduced to sitting after a period of bedrest, it is important that a schedule is established that slowly increases the time that they sit out according to their skin tolerance.

Pressure-relieving equipment

The use of pressure-relieving equipment is necessary for those patients at risk and for anyone with established pressure damage. The type of equipment will depend on the patient's mobility, degree of risk and availability within the care setting.

There is a vast array of equipment commercially available, which can make appropriate selection confusing. Most of the equipment available has not been reliably evaluated and no best buy can be recommended (Cullum *et al*, 2004). This equipment will range from pressure reducing foam mattresses for at-risk patients, to alternating air overlays and mattress replacements systems for patients at higher risk. Very complex low air loss or air fluidised systems may be required for critically ill patients. Electric profiling beds have been shown to be effective in both patient positioning and pressure reduction. Simply gatching the knees can result in a reduction in pressure on the sacrum and heels (Gray *et al*, 2001; Keogh and Dealey, 2001). Electric beds can result in improved mobility by the patient who may find it easier to get in and out of bed when the bed height is adjustable. Decisions on equipment selection should be based on the overall assessment of the patient, including skin inspection and not on the score generated from a risk assessment scale.

Table 4.3 shows some of the issues that need to be considered when selecting equipment.

Equipment selection flowcharts are often used to assist in decision making.

Table 4.3: Pressure-relieving equipment considerations
Does the patient find it comfortable?
Is the equipment in good working order, eg. cover intact?
Do I know how to use this equipment, especially in an emergency?
Do I know how to clean and decontaminate this equipment?
Do I know where the instructions are?
Is this equipment suitable for the weight of the patient?
Has the equipment been adjusted for the weight of the patient?
If the patient is sitting out, have seating requirements been considered?
Is the chair the correct height for the patient?
Has the use of equipment been documented in the patient's notes?

Management of established pressure ulcers

It is essential to recognise the first signs of pressure damage and to act immediately. The first priority is to relieve any pressure from the affected area and limit any further damage. The basic components of your preventative plan such as skin care, positioning and nutrition will need to continued and monitored and alterations made is necessary.

> *Patient scenario five*
>
> What type of pressure relieving equipment would be suitable for Mr Skelton? What factors will you take into consideration when making your decision?
>
> Equipment:
>
> Factors:

Grading ulcers

The degree of damage will need to be determined. Grading scales are available that will assist in classifying this damage. This information is useful as part of the overall wound management and will assist in monitoring progress. It is advisable to photograph the pressure ulcer. The grade of ulcer may change as healing takes place. In some instances, the grade may increase as debridement takes place and the full extent of the injury becomes apparent. There are a variety of grading scales available, some being more complex than others. A study by Russell and Reynolds (2001) showed that the use of a simpler score resulted in more consistent recordings. The European Pressure Ulcer Advisory Panel grading scale is shown in *Appendix 3*. Grading scales should be used to determine the initial extent of the damage. They should not be used in reverse, ie. in the assessment of tissue repair (NPUAP, 1995).

Wound management

The basic principles of wound assessment and management will need to be incorporated in the care of a patient with pressure damage (see sections on wound assessment and management). Common challenges have been identified and include the following (Dunford, 1998):

⌘ Debridement of necrotic and sloughy tissue.
⌘ Control of exudate and accompanying odour.
⌘ Grade 3 and 4 ulcers may present as cavity wounds. These will require the use of cavity fillers and dressings or the use of vacuum-assisted wound closure.
⌘ Pressure ulcers commonly occur on the sacrum and heels. The proximity of the sacrum to the anus and the narrowness of the heel often make them difficult to dress. The use of adhesive dressings or dressings cut to size will allow more flexibility.
⌘ Pressure ulcers can cause significant pain, which is often under-estimated and can result in an increase in stress levels, social isolation and disturbed sleep.

Patient scenario six

Once again look at Mr Skelton's pressure ulcer shown in *Figure 2.7*. Can you grade this ulcer using the EPUAP grading scale shown in the appendices?

Grade:

The role of nutrition

Nutrition plays an important role both in the prevention and management of pressure ulceration. Although poor nutritional status may not be a major causal factor in itself, it is a contributing factor in the development of pressure ulcer (McLaren and Green, 2001; Mathus-Vliegen, 2001). Studies have indicated that the nutritional status of both hospital and community-based patients with pressure ulcers is poor (Lewis, 1996; Strauss and Maargolis, 1996; Green *et al*, 1999) with deficiencies in protein, vitamin C and zinc, which are all vital for wound healing. Defiencies may be even greater if there is a high exudate loss from the ulcer.

Identification of malnutrition is vital for both the prevention and management of pressure ulcers. Visual assessment of skin areas, regular weighing and calculation of body mass index (BMI), together with nutritionally specific questions regarding ability to eat and any unintentional weight loss will all assist in detecting problems at an early stage (Russell, 2000).

If malnutrition is apparent, then either increased dietary intake or supplementation will be required before wound healing will become established. Dietary input should be approximately 30/35 cal/kg/day and 1.25–1.5 grams of protein/kg/day to re-establish a positive nitrogen balance (AHCPR, 1994). The elderly have higher requirements of protein than the recommended daily allowance (RDA) of 0.8 g/kg which is not often appreciated (Mathus-Vliegen, 2001). Repeat assessments, including measurement of serum albumin to detect protein levels, should be used to evaluate nutritional support.

Prevention of recurrence

Once a pressure ulcer has healed, it is important to prevent recurrence, especially as the resultant scar tissue will have a reduced tensile strength. It is important that patients and carers fully understand how pressure ulcers develop and any actions that should be taken if problems occur. The best management strategies will be rendered useless if changes are not made to the environment in which pressure ulceration has occurred, otherwise further ulceration could develop (Dunford, 1998).

Key points

❖ Pressure ulcers are caused by prolonged or high levels or pressure combined with other variables such as shear, friction and moisture.

❖ It is often the combination of these that leads to tissue distortion and destruction.

❖ The most important factors in preventing pressure ulcers are to identify those who are at risk and to alleviate the forces that cause pressure damage.

❖ Good skin care, keeping the patient mobile and addressing nutritional needs are all essential in the prevention and treatment of pressure ulcers and also to prevent recurrence once healed.

❖ Pressure-relieving equipment is required for patients at risk and with established skin damage. Seating requirements will also need consideration and should include the length of time a patient is sat out together with the need for specialist chairs and cushions.

Leg ulceration

Definition

Leg ulcers have been defined as 'an area of discontinuity of epidermis or dermis on the lower legs or feet, persisting for six weeks or more' (Dale *et al*, 1983). Although this definition includes the whole of the lower leg, in practice, ulcers of the feet are often further defined. For example, a 'black heel' may be classed as a pressure ulcer.

Epidemiology

Estimates on the prevalence of leg ulceration in the UK vary: 1.8 per 1000 (Cornwall *et al*, 1986), 2.4 per 1000 (Vickery *et al*, 1999), 2.8 per 1000 (Moffatt *et al*, 1992). The incidence of leg ulceration increases with age, especially for women and it is estimated that 1–2% of the population will develop a leg ulcer at some time in their lives (Morison and Moffat, 1994). Socio-economic factors have also been found to contribute to morbidity. A London study found that a lower social class, single status and lack of central heating significantly reduced healing rates (Franks *et al*, 1995).

Costs

The financial costs of managing leg ulceration are considerable. To the cost of dressings must be added that of nursing time, usually of district nurses but also, to a lesser extent, practice nurses, who provide the bulk of leg ulcer care. A recent Cornish study found that for that county, with a population of 432,248, the 1998 costs of treating leg ulcers in the community was £835,735.85 (Vickery *et al*, 1999). Even a decade ago, total NHS costs were estimated at a possible £400 million a year (Laing,1992)

In human terms, the cost of having a leg ulcer is also great. Pain, sleeplessness, social isolation and reduced mobility significantly impact of life quality. While these factors are profound, it is often the more noticeable factors such as odour and leakage that cause the most distress because they can be apparent to others (Walshe, 1995).

Causes

It has been estimated that underlying venous disease is responsible for between 70–75% of all leg ulcers in the UK, with 8–10% caused by arterial disease (Collier, 1996). Another 10–15% will have mixed venous and arterial components (Morison and Moffat, 1994).

Other less common causes, accounting in total for a further 2–5% include: malignancy, trauma, blood disorders, metabolic disorders and dermatological problems.

Diabetes mellitus and rheumatoid arthritis require a special mention. These are systemic disorders which affect many biochemical and metabolic processes within the body. Their presence may precipitate ulcer formation and prevent healing in a number of ways. The main one being the damaging affects these diseases can have on the blood vessels, particularly those in the peripheries. The body's ability to deliver oxygenated blood to the lower limb may be reduced. These two conditions may well co-exist with each other and with other disorders leading to leg ulcer formation. They may generally be regarded as exacerbating factors, rather than primary causes in their own right, although their hindering affects on the progress of an ulcer may be severe.

The main types of leg ulcers

Venous ulcers

The function of the heart is to pump blood out on the arterial side on its journey to the peripheries. However, the venous side has no corresponding heart-like structure to propel blood along the return journey. Instead, this side relies on the squeezing effect that the powerful muscles of the calf have on the deep veins of the leg. As the muscles contract, the veins are compressed flat, this has the effect of pushing the returning blood along and up. As the muscle relaxes, eg. between paces, the veins refill with more blood, ready likewise to be moved on during the next phase of muscle contraction. This mechanism is known as the calf muscle pump.

To prevent the blood going in the wrong direction or simply falling back and pooling in the legs, the veins, unlike arteries, have valves. The valves consist of flap-like structures, which freely permit blood through on its return to the heart, but close to prevent back-flow.

Just as the arterial system relies on the health and good functioning of the heart to perform well, so too does the venous system rely on the health of the calf muscle pump and the valves. Any diseases or injuries or other conditions which significantly impede the action of these mechanisms will ultimately affect the health of the leg.

Reasons for poor valve performance may include congenital or familial defect, damage from previous deep vein thrombosis, surgery or injury and mechanical failure due to a higher obstruction to the venous return. This can be caused by obesity whereby a prominent abdomen can occlude vessels in the groin. Regular chair sleeping combined with poor mobility can also significantly impair venous return leading to the condition known as 'armchair leg'. Reasons for calf muscle pump failure include poor mobility, even when mobility appears generally adequate good gait is essential. Injuries and diseases which limit the range of movement within the ankle joint, will ultimately impinge on the performance of the calf muscle pump.

If one or both of these mechanisms are sufficiently under performing, blood flow becomes sluggish and there is pooling of fluid within the tissues. This oedema slows down gaseous exchange within the microcirculation; the tissues are less well oxygenated and toxins not adequately removed. Eventually, tissue health suffers and skin lesions appear often without an additional insult such as a knock or a scratch. To the sufferer who may well be unaware of the underlying disease process, these lesions appear to have no apparent cause. Patients often state being unaware of a problem until they notice staining on socks or stockings and find they have the beginnings of an ulcer.

Arterial ulcers

In addition to good functioning of the heart, the arterial system also relies on the health of the vessels. Diseases such as diabetes and hypertension and other degenerative disorders allow the accumulation of plaques, cells and other debris which narrows the lumen of the vessels, obstructing blood flow (Phillips, 1996). Cigarette smoke contains substances which cause vasoconstriction (narrowing of the blood vessel walls), therefore smoking can seriously exacerbate an existing problem. Poor blood flow means reduced oxygenation of the tissues and accumulation of toxins, particularly at the peripheries. Eventually ulcers occur.

Mixed ulcers

It is very common for both the above vascular problems to be present in the same individual. Indeed, both conditions may even be present and the ulceration actually due to a third cause. A careful assessment of all leg ulcers should be undertaken by a competent practitioner to establish exactly what the problem is. Examples of venous and arterial leg ulcers are shown in *Figures 4.5* and *4.6*.

Chronic oedema

Prompt intervention to reverse or reduce the pathophysiological (disease processes within the body) changes that occur within the tissues of the leg, subsequent to venous disease, can increase ulcer healing rates and avoid the development of chronic oedema. Chronic oedema is defined as swelling of greater than three months' duration, which does not resolve on elevation. If developing oedema is left unchecked eventually profound, often irreversible, tissue changes can occur. This is as a result of excessive hydrostatic pressure, reduced oxygenation and the accumulation of waste products which are irritant. The tissues become chronically inflamed and fibrosed with an increase in subcutaneous fat. The skin can become hyperkeratotic (scaly and dry) and other skin lesions develop such as papillomatosis (giving the skin a cobblestone appearance). Skin creases occur. Often these are very deep and provide a moist environment for the development of fungal infections.

A longstanding excessive load of extra fluid within the tissues will eventually overload the lymphatic system, reducing local capacity to return lymph to the circulation, thus further exacerbating the problem. One major effect of this disease process for tissue viability practitioners is the resulting increased risk of infection due to the impairment of the immune surveillance capability of the lymphatic system. Good skin care and patient education to reduce the risk of additional trauma are essential mainstays in management.

Assessment

Treatment for leg ulceration fundamentally depends on the cause, therefore the assessment underpins correct treatment. If, for example, the treatment for venous ulceration were applied to arterial ulcers there would at best be ineffective treatment and, at worse, disastrous life-threatening consequences. This is because the treatment for venous ulcers is the complete antithesis of that for arterial ones.

A full clinical history and physical examination is required (RCN Guidelines, 1998). Factors suggesting venous disease include:

- family history of venous disease, eg. varicose veins
- presence of varicose veins whether treated or not
- history of deep vein thrombosis

- history of phlebitis
- previous surgery or trauma to the affected leg.

Factors suggestive of other aetiology, include:

- history of heart disease, stroke, transient ischaemic attack
- diabetes mellitus
- peripheral vascular disease/intermittent claudication
- cigarette smoking
- rheumatoid arthritis

Other past medical history and information on other current problems experienced or being treated for, eg. tiredness, weight loss or gain, changes in mood should be noted. A list of current medication should be recorded.

Baseline measurements should include a urine test, particularly for; glucose, height, weight, pulse and blood pressure, ankle and calf measurements.

An examination of the ulcer should include its size, shape, site, appearance, with enquiry about duration and treatments tried. Also, if there has been any previous ulcers together with treatments used.

Physical examination should also include the physical appearance of the lower limb, noting the presence or absence of oedema, scars, other skin problems such as eczema, haemosiderin staining (dark brown pigmentation around the gaiter area), pedal pulses and general foot perfusion.

A careful history taking of pain; its type, onset, what exacerbates or relieves it, the effectiveness or otherwise of analgesics, is a particularly useful indicator as to ulcer type.

The practitioner should observe for themselves what is demonstrable, eg. the degree of mobility exhibited, gait pattern, level of understanding about the problem. A record should also be made about social and lifestyle issues, such as; housing, nutrition, if stairs are used, if patient lives alone, who cooks and cleans, if the patient sleeps in a bed and if the patient smokes. The practitioner should also elicit from the patient their worries, concerns and wishes about the leg ulcer which may often, surprisingly, be very different indeed from that of the practitioner. For example, the lady with a severely ischaemic foot who doesn't want surgery because she is worried about who would look after her dog if she were in hospital.

Doppler assessment

A final but essential part of the assessment is that of Doppler ultrasound to establish the ankle brachial pressure index (ABPI). For this test the patient should be rested and, ideally, lying flat. The pressure of the ankle pulses are recorded using a hand-held Doppler ultrasound. Some practitioners aim to obtain all four (posterial tibial, peroneal, anterior tibial and dorsalis pedis), but it is recommended that at least two are found (Vowden, 1998; Davies, 2001) (excluding the combination of anterior tibial and dorsalis pedis, the latter being an extension of the former). The highest of the readings for each leg is used to calculate the ABPI. Similarly, both brachial pressures are recorded. The higher of the two brachial readings is taken to establish the ABPI. For each leg the calculable ankle reading is divided by the brachial reading.

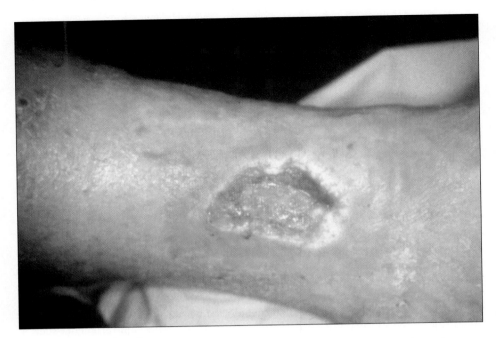

Figure 4.5: Venous leg ulcer

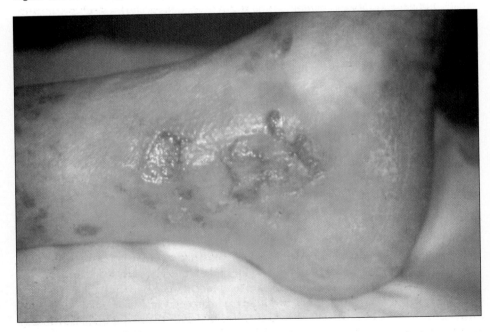

Figure 4.6: Arterial leg ulcer

In normal health, the ankle pressures are the same as or greater than the brachial pressures (Davies, 2001), which will give a reading of 1.0 or >1.0. If there is a reduced flow of blood to the limb, the reading will be < 1.0. It is recommended that patients with readings of <0.8 should be referred for vascular assessment (RCN Guidelines, 1998).

Treatment

Following all the formal processes of assessment the practitioner is in a position to decide the likely cause of the ulcer and appropriate treatment can begin.

If the patient has been assessed as having a venous problem and the **ABPI is 0.8 or greater**, the standard treatment is compression (RCN Guidelines, 1998). This is applied either through hosiery, if the ulcer is small enough, or through bandaging. There is some doubt as to how and why compression actually works. One assumption is that compression supports the damaged valves for them to perform more effectively, thereby improving venous return and reducing oedema. Another theory is that compression has more effect on the micro rather than the macrocirculation (large vessels). One suggestion has been that whether veins are damaged or not, the ultimate situation is that of raised hydrostatic pressure which compression reverses (Rees, 2002). Whatever the underlying mechanism, compression can achieve significant healing rates (Vowden *et al*, 2000).

There are two main compression bandage system types, short-stretch and long-stretch. Long-stretch bandages have a high resting pressure and a low working pressure and short-stretch bandages have a high working pressure and a low resting pressure. Long-stretch bandages are considered most useful in patients with reduced mobility and, while short-stretch bandages can be used in patients with venous ulceration, they are used exclusively along with hosiery in the management of lymphoedema.

Changes in the drug tariff have resulted in various compression bandaging systems becoming available in the community (Vowden *et al*, 2000). Long-stretch systems first became available in 1998 as a kit form and were known as the Charing Cross four-layer (or multi-layer) system. Their use was widely adopted following a large study demonstrating their effectiveness, led by Christine Moffatt (Moffat and Dickson, 1993).

Assessing for and applying compression bandages is a highly skilled activity and should only be performed by someone competent to do so. Selection of the appropriate system takes account of factors such as ankle size, lifestyle, if infection is present and therefore more frequent viewing of the ulcer bed is required, who will perform the bandaging and economics (some bandages can be washed and reused).

The bandages are applied from toe to knee and a wool or wadding bandage layer is always placed beneath the compression layers to prevent pressure damage. The method of application varies with different systems and is in accordance with the manufacturer's instructions.

Ulcers of whatever suggested aetiology in which the ABPI is <0.8, should be referred for a vascular opinion and compression not applied. If the problem is clearly arterial an urgent referral may be needed. Likewise, suspected malignant ulcers, ulcers in patients with poorly managed diabetes or rheumatoid arthritis, should have appropriate specialist referrals.

Dressings

The choice of dressing for venous ulcers will be based on the same criteria as for any wound with some slight modification. This is because compression itself is ultimately the treatment for venous ulceration not the dressing. In addition, the bandage layers themselves have the potential to maintain the warm, moist environment required for healing. Simple, low adherent dressings are recommended (RCN Guidelines, 1998).

Leg ulcers, especially those on the feet of patients with marked ischaemia, should be kept dry. In the presence of poor perfusion healing will be prolonged and the immune system less effective. Therefore, maintaining a moist, warm environment, which permits microorganisms to flourish, could lead to life-threatening infection.

Surgical options

Arterial problems are always more serious than venous ones as without an adequate blood supply to an area, tissue death will quickly occur. Angiograpy, whereby a radio-opaque dye is injected into the arteries proximal to the problem area and images recorded of its progress may be required to locate the blockage. If the problem is due to a discrete blockage then angioplasty is often possible, whereby the affected vessel is dilated and the blockage removed. More extensive blockages may require graft or bypass surgery to create an adequate flow, which are altogether more complex procedures.

In venous disease, if the problem lies within the deep veins then surgery is not an option. Problems within the superficial and perforator veins may be amenable to surgery. In these cases the damaged section may be removed or otherwise isolated from the venous system.

> *Time out*
>
> Imagine you are a patient with a newly diagnosed venous leg ulcer and have just been told that you have to wear several layers of tight bandaging over your very sore ulcer. What do you think your thoughts would be? List some of the practical problems and economic costs that you might foresee.

Patient education

In every sphere of nursing activity, patient education is central to a successful outcome. In the management of venous leg ulceration good patient education assumes an even greater importance. This is because the treatment being suggested may appear counter intuitive to the patient. They ask themselves how can a tight thick bandage on my sore, painful leg possibly help? Surely I need something soft and cosy? Their preoccupation and belief is in the choice of dressing, that the dressing will heal the wound. They are surprised at the lack of emphasis to this area of care. Furthermore, they are sometimes bewildered by the sheer amount of bandage and dressing material used. They may have an ulcer the size of a 5 pence piece, on the inner aspect of the ankle, that could easily be covered up with a flesh coloured island dressing, so they find it ludicrous to be told that a large bulky set of bandages must go from toe to knee.

The practitioner needs to anticipate these questions and provide clear and adequate answers. Practical problems may include not being able to wear usual footwear or close fitting trousers or being able to drive a car safely. The prospect of weekly bandage changes impinges on normal lifestyle and may be severely restricting. General skin care of the leg, as opposed to the wound, is also important and the patient's leg should be washed with an emollient such as Aqeuous Cream and further emollient applied when the leg has been dried. By arrangement, the patient may be encouraged to bath or shower prior to the reapplication of bandages, with the proviso that not too long is spent without bandages in place.

Support and advice to overcome these difficulties and appreciate the need for treatment should be ongoing. Once patients can begin to see improvements for themselves the going gets easier, but initial compliance often depends on the successful interpersonal skills and practising style of the individual practitioner.

National guidelines

National clinical practice guidelines on the management of patients with venous leg ulcers have been available since 1998 and are now available in full version on the Internet and can be readily downloaded. The guidelines should be the basis for all leg ulcer management and are essential reading for anyone wishing to practice in this area.

Key points

❖ Leg ulceration is a painful common problem, especially for women which increases with age and is exacerbated by immobility.

❖ Leg ulcers can have various causes, the most common being venous disease, whereby oedema, skin changes and staining around the gaiter area are often present.

❖ The mainstay in the treatment of venous leg ulceration is compression, either in the form of bandages or hosiery.

❖ Assessment and management of leg ulceration requires additional skills.

Diabetic foot ulceration

Diabetes mellitus is a chronic metabolic disorder characterised by a disturbance in glucose homeostasis, which often leads to vascular and neurological changes predisposing to a higher level of morbidity (King, 2003). It is estimated to affect around 3% of the population of the United Kingdom (Foster, 2000).

Definition

Diabetic foot ulcers are mainly caused by a combination of three factors:

- peripheral neuropathy
- peripheral arterial disease
- mechanical abnormalities of the foot (Brill *et al*, 1997).

However, other morbidity associated with diabetes, eg. previous amputation and visual and mobility problems do increase risk (Scottish Intercollegiate Guidelines Network, [SIGN] 2001).

Epidemiology

In the United Kingdom the prevalence of foot ulceration in persons with diabetes is about 5–7% (SIGN Guidelines, 2001) which is estimated to be fifteen times higher than for the general population (Bild *et al*, 1989)

Costs to the patient and society

Expenditure on diabetes was estimated in 1997 to account for approximately 9% of the total NHS budget (Currie *et al*, 1997), with foot ulceration as the commonest reason for hospital admission for patients with diabetes (Young *et al*, 1994). Economic costs are associated with nursing and medical care and with treatments such as dressings, but there are also huge indirect costs in terms of reduced earning potential, reduced quality of life, increased incidence of disability, infection and social isolation.

Causes

In diabetes the regulation of glucose within the body is disturbed. This may result in extended periods of high blood glucose levels (hyperglycaemia). If the high glucose levels are poorly regulated, nerves, blood vessels, bone and other structures within the tissues, especially at the peripheries, become irreversibly damaged. This excess of glucose is the cause, directly or indirectly, of all the other problems.

Key proteins in nerve tissue become glucolysated (degraded by the glucose), which interferes with their function (Brill *et al*, 1997). Both motor and sensory nerves are affected. Damage to sensory nerves reduces the person's capacity to appreciate pain. The person may be oblivious to the onset of ulceration because they cannot feel it. Diabetic retinopathy (damage to the retina) may also mean that they cannot see an ulcer, allowing it to develop unnoticed. Conversely, damage to the nerves may have the opposite effect, whereby there is abnormal sensation or increased pain. An example of a diabetic foot ulcer with obvious sensory nerve damage is shown in *Figure 4.6*.

Damage to the motor nerves activating the muscles of the foot leads to changes in the architecture of the foot. The person's gait and the distribution of pressure across the foot are affected leading to pressure 'hot spots'. Callous is laid down in these areas of high pressure in an attempt by the body to avoid tissue damage. If there is no relief from the increased pressure, eg. by removal of callous and by modifiying footwear, eventually the stresses become so great that tissue does break down.

The autonomic nerves are also affected. This results in unopposed vasodilation with a higher than normal blood flow through bone, which is poorly tolerated. Bone becomes soft, leading to fractures and distortion which further affect the foot's architecture. In severe cases the pedal arch collapses, a condition known as 'Charcot's foot' (Larsen *et al*, 2001).

It should be remembered that the foot is a highly complex, strong and flexible structure which depends upon an intact framework of small bones and ligaments, muscles and nerves. The effects of the chemical activity of glucose over a long period stiffen joints, waste muscle and degrade bone, and eventually deformity becomes inevitable.

Even the skin of the foot is affected. The impairment of the autonomic nerves regulating the skin's ability to breathe and sweat result in an increased dryness and tendency to crack, reducing resistance to injury (Brill *et al*, 1997).

Once damage has occurred, impairment of leucocyte function, also through hyperglycaemia, inhibits the body's ability to fight infection. Once infection gets a hold, an ulcer may quickly increase in size and become a life-threatening problem unless managed correctly.

The effects of hyperglycaemia on the microcirculation of a person with diabetes also increases their risk of developing peripheral vascular disease (Brill *et al*, 1997). Persons with diabetes are four times as likely to develop the condition. Atherosclerotic plaques build up reducing the lumen size of vessels until they eventually occlude. The foot becomes increasingly at risk through ischaemia. Necrosis (tissue death) can occur and amputation may be the only option.

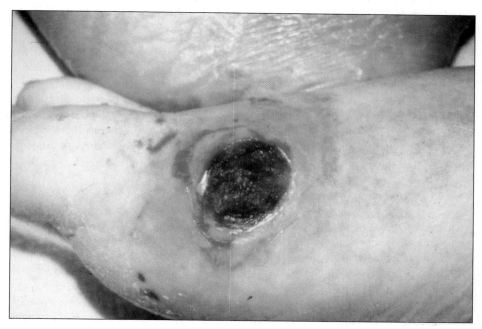

Figure 4.6: Neuropathic foot ulcer

Prevention

The diabetic foot is vulnerable to damage or injury from even a minor insult. Ill-fitting footwear, burns from hot water bottles, cold injuries and neglected nails have all led to incidence of foot ulceration. Patients should be encouraged to check their shoes before putting them on (to ensure coins or other items have not inadvertently fallen which will not be perceived by the feet). Feet should be inspected regularly for callus or sore areas and, if present, their presence should be reported to whoever provides the patients on-going foot care. Patients should also be advised not to walk with bare feet, especially outdoors, to protect from cold and heat and to wear well-fitting socks without raised seams in addition to well-fitting shoes. Dryness of the skin can be reduced by using appropriate moisturising foot creams.

Time out

The management of diabetic foot ulceration is a multidisciplinary activity. Which professionals (and which non-professional) do you think may best contribute to providing optimum care?

Treatment options

There are three mainstays of treatment for diabetic foot ulceration:

- good wound management
- off-loading of pressure
- control of infection.

However, management will founder if the patient is not thoroughly educated and committed to a disciplined programme of foot care. The patient should be regarded as a central member of the team.

The bedrock of good management depends on thorough and ongoing assessment, not only of the feet but also of the patient's general health including glucose control and of the patient's lifestyle, eg. diet and smoking. Diabetes is an insiduous disease affecting the whole body. In order to maximise the potential for wound healing, the health of the whole body must be considered.

Wound management

The management of the diabetic foot ulcer is very different to general wound management. Because of the high risk of infection and the increased speed at which infection can get a hold, together with altered sensation whereby the patient has lost the protective pain response, the ulcer must be inspected more often than ordinary wounds (Foster, 2000).

Moist wound healing is advocated for the majority of wounds. If the wound is necrotic or sloughy the moisture will aid the break down of dead tissue. Moist wounds attract bacteria which the natural body defences normally prevent becoming a problem. In a patient with diabetes those defences are compromised: although moist wound healing is not outlawed, it requires very skilled supervision. Practitioners, while not drying out the ulcer entirely, often prefer to keep it slightly drier than they would a non-diabetic ulcer. For this reason, occlusive dressings are often avoided and there is more use of sharp rather than chemical debridement. Necrotic tissue and slough are removed much quicker by this method, reducing the opportunity for infection to get established. Sharp debridement must always be performed by a practitioner trained in this procedure.

Off-loading of pressure

Footwear for people with diabetes should always be well-fitting with the toe box both deep and wide enough to accommodate the foot adequately. Where actual ulceration has occurred, pressure over the damaged area must be removed to allow the ulcer to heal. Orthotic inserts may be required or, in more serious cases, orthotic boots or casts are used. Where adequate off-loading cannot be achieved by other means, strict bedrest may be the only option.

Control of infection

As feet are naturally in contact with the ground, any ulcerated areas should be well covered with robust dressings and changed when 'strike through' occurs. This reduces the opportunity for bacteria to gain access. Antibacterial dressings may be used either alone or in conjunction with other dressings. Because of the high risk of recurrent infections, the diabetic foot ulcer is one of the few wounds where prophylactic use of antibacterial dressings and oral antibiotics should be considered.

Regular and frequent inspection of the ulcer and the foot in general for signs of clinical infection is essential. The ulcer is likely to be colonised anyway, therefore a wound swab should only be taken when evidence of infection is present. Antibiotics should be commenced immediately and the choice of preparation reviewed on receipt of the culture and sensitivity. There is much concern nowadays about the over- and inappropriate prescribing of antibiotics, especially in the management of wounds such as leg and pressure ulcers. However, the consequences of failing to prescribe adequate and timely antibiotic therapy for the diabetic foot ulcer can have dire consequences.

Key points

❖   Diabetes is a multifactorial systemic disease leading to various pathologies.

❖   The management of the diabetic foot should be regarded as a multi-disciplinary activity, often requiring the combined skills of the patient, the nurse, the podiatrist, the orthotist, the diabetologist and the physiotherapist.

❖   Diabetic ulceration of the feet can be largely prevented by assiduous attention to care of the feet and the avoidance of foot injury.

Burns

It has been estimated that 150 000 new patients will attend A&E departments each year with burn injuries (Wardrope and Edhouse, 1998). Unfortunately, a high percentage of these will be children. In 1999, 47,000 children in the UK sustained a burn or scald (Taylor, 2001). Serious burns are less common than minor burns and despite major, national fire prevention campaigns they still remain a significant cause of death and serious injury.

The degree of tissue destruction following a burn is directly related both to the temperature and the duration of exposure to the heat source. Following burn injury, changes continue to occur in the affected tissue for some time and significant tissue damage can occur some time after the initial insult (Richard, 1998).

Burn injuries have three specific zones:

⌘ Coagulation – the area of non-viable tissue which is at the centre of the burn.
⌘ Stasis – the tissue is viable but fragile and at high risk due to reduced tissue perfusion.
⌘ Hyperaemia – this is the area surrounding the burn which will also be involved in the inflammatory process but the tissue is intact.

Sources of burn injuries are shown in *Table 4.4*.

Table 4.4: Sources of burn injuries	
Type of burn	**Common examples**
Wet heat (scalds)	Steam, domestic accidents involving hot drinks, boiling water, hot baths or hot oils
Dry heat	Contact with flame or hot surfaces
Chemical	Acid or alkali from chemcals, batteries
Electrical	Domestic or industrial (power lines) or lightening
Radiation	UV light (sunburn, sunlamps)
Intense cold	Exposure to liquid nitrogen

First aid for burns

The first priority following any burn injury is to ensure the safety of the patient using the ABC of trauma management (airway, breathing, circulation). There may well be a compromised airway and pulmonary complications following the inhalation of smoke or fumes. Following this, first aid treatment for the burn should take place. Irrigation with clean, cool water for between ten to twenty minutes is the recommended treatment, as this will dissipate heat and prevent further damage and limit the zone of stasis. The one exception to water irrigation is, in the case of burns with metallic sodium, potassium and calcium, all of which react with water (Atkinson, 1998). Clothes that are soaked in hot liquid or burnt on should be carefully removed (ETRS guidelines, 1999). It is highly likely that the person involved will be very distressed so support and reassurance will be needed.

Dressings should not be applied before the burn is properly assessed; however, cling film applied loosely is an ideal temporary dressing. Any tight, restrictive clothing should be removed so as not to cause constrictions and, if possible, the area of the body elevated to reduce oedema which is a natural consequence following a burn injury. Tetanus prophylaxis should also be considered.

Time out

For your own protection against burn injury, are you aware of the rules for safe sunbathing? What advice would you give to a parent with young children concerning this?

Assessment of burns

❖ *Extent of the burn (body surface area)*

There are several methods of assessing the body surface area (BSA) of burn injury. These include the Rule of Nines, which divides the body into percentage areas for a gross estimate of the extent of burn injury. The Lund-Browder method is similar and provides a more precise estimation. The palm method of assessment will also provide a rough estimate of BSA, as the palm of the patient's hand with fingers closed is considered equivalent to 1% of the BSA.

Establishing the extent of the burn will also assist in classifying the severity of the injury. Burns covering more than 15% of an adult's body surface or 10% in the case of a child, may require immediate intravenous fluid resuscitation in a burns unit and are classified as major burns. A burn of less than 5% in an adult which does not require a skin graft, is classified as minor. Others are classified as intermediate (Atkinson, 1998). Burns involving the head, face, hands or perineum will also require specialist treatment.

❖ *Depth of the burn*

The various depths of burn together with presentation and treatment options are shown in *Table 4.5*. In most cases a degree of clinical judgement is required as many burns will not fit into clear cut categories and may not be of uniform depth. The burn injury is also prone to changes in appearance within the first few days (Richard, 1999).

Additional considerations for burn injuries

❖ *Blisters*

Blisters are caused by a separation of the epidermis and dermis due to the accumulation of tissue fluid between the layers (Tortora and Grabowski, 2000). The management of blisters remains controversial; however, the general consensus is to leave blisters intact where possible and to allow a gradual absorption of blister fluid (Flanagan and Graham, 2001). Blisters can be covered with a semi-permeable film dressing to add protection. If it is not possible to leave the blisters intact, a suitable occlusive or semi-occlusive dressing should be used in order to maintain a moist environment.

❖ *Nutritional needs*

The body will enter a hypermetabolic state following burn injury which will result in increased energy requirements. A high calorie and high protein diet will be required in order to compensate for this (Regojo, 2003).

Table 4.5: Classification of burns

Depth of burn	Skin involved	Presentation	Treatment options
Superficial, ie. sunburn	Epidermis only	Skin is pink/red and tender/painful. Usually dry and no blisters. Minmal risk of infection	3–5 days to heal Emollients Calamine, after sun lotions
Superficial partial thickness	Epidermis and superficial dermis	Skin is bright pink/red. Blanches with brisk capillary refill when pressure is applied. Blisters present and surface moist. Very painful (exposed nerve endings)	10–21 days to heal. Will require dressings to maintain moist healing environment (low -adherent silicone, hydrocolloid foam or film dressings). Possible changes in skin pigmentation but scarring not usually problem
Deep partial thickness	Epidermis and dermis	Skin red/waxy white. Blanches with slow capillary refill. Skin may have altered sensation or be insensate (nerve endings destroyed). Wet and oedematous, possibly large blisters. Rapid heat and fluid loss	14–21 days to heal through formation of granulation and epithelialization. Will require skin grafting in order to limit scarring. Topical antimicrobials agents may be used together with dressings to ensure a moist healing environment
Full thickness	Epidermis and dermis destroyed. Fascia, muscle and bone may	Skin leathery, dry, possibly charred and white (totally ischaemic), beige brown or black (necrotic). Not painful except edges (nerves intact here) oedematous	Weeks–months to heal. Excise deep skin and apply skin grafts or skin equivalents. Topical antimicrobial agents for infection risk. Prone to contracture formation and scarring. Pressure garments may be required

adapted from Regojo, 2003; Richard, 1999; Fowler, 1999

❖ **Infection risk**

Burns will suppress the immune system and so increase the risk of infection. Careful observation for signs of infection is important and the use of antimicrobial agents (eg. silver sulphadiazine) may be required.

It is also important to debride all non-viable skin as quickly as possible

❖ **Skin care**

The use of emollients will be required on healed areas, together with a high factor sunscreen. Scars may require specialist management, such as the use of gel sheets and pressure garments.

❖ **Pain**

Burns are extremely painful due to exposed nerve endings. Anxiety can also heighten any pain, which may be increased with the prospect of dressing changes. This pain needs to be thoroughly assessed using a suitable pain assessment chart and appropriate analgesia given. This is particularly important in the case of children where the use of needles for analgesic delivery would increase their distress. Suitable analgesics in this case may include oral morphine sulphate, intranasal diamorphine, paracetamol or Entonox® (Taylor, 2001). Careful selection of wound care products, such as the use of silicone products, can also reduce pain (*Chapter 3, pp. 26–29*). The patient and their family should be fully involved in their care at each stage to help reduce anxiety.

❖ *Emotional aftercare*

Patients who have had burn injuries may suffer psychosocial distress for which support will be required. Counselling and support networks such as Changing Faces may help them adapt to any altered body image and the distress of the event (Dearden *et al*, 2001).

Key points

❖ The first aid treatment of burns involves the ABC of trauma management, irrigation with clean, cool water for ten to twenty minutes followed by the application of a temporary clean dressing.

❖ There are several methods of assessing the body surface area (BSA) of burn injury. These include the Rule of Nines and the Lund-Browder method. The depth of burn also needs assessing and may range from superficial, partial thickness to full thickness.

❖ Additional considerations of burn injuries include infection risk, increased nutritional demands, pain management, skin care and emotional support and aftercare.

Malignant and fungating wounds

Definition

Malignant wounds are areas of malignant growth and ulceration. Infiltration of malignant cells into the skin and supporting structures can result in a fungating tumour. These are often described as 'fungus–like' or 'cauliflower-like' because of their appearance. Initially, they may present as nodules that then break down into ulcerated areas. Each presentation is quite unique and they vary significantly in their appearance and size (Grocott, 1999). The fungating wound can result from a local primary source or as a result of metastatic spread (Grocott, 1999).They are often associated with advanced cancer, particularly carcinoma of the breast (Adderley and Smith, 2002). An example of an extensive fungating breast wound is shown in *Figure 4.8*.

Squamous cell carcinomas can also develop in chronic wounds, often those of long standing, and are referred to as Marjolin's ulcers (Akguner *et al*, 1998). The presence of Marjolin ulcers are confirmed following a wound biopsy, which should always be considered when there are any unusual changes to the wound and presentations such as exudate, pain and appearance (Naylor, 2002).

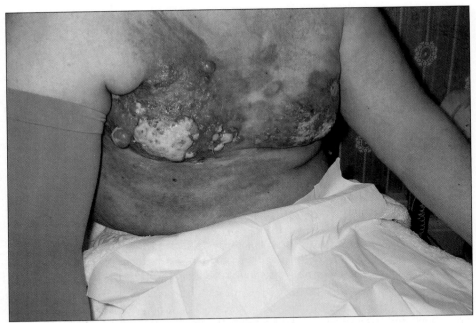

Figure 4.8: Fungating breast wound, courtesy of Patricia Grocott

Size of problem

The prevalence of malignant and fungating wounds is unknown and they remain relatively rare. A study by Haisfield-Wolfe and Rund (1997) estimated that 5–10% of patients with metastatic cancer will develop such a wound. The most common presentation is the breast, although they can also occur on the head, face and neck and the perineum and genitalia.

Presenting problems

The malignant cells can be very prolific and interfere with tissue oxygentation, lymphatic drainage and haemostasis (Adderley and Smith, 2002). Necrotic tissue can occur due to the reduced tissue perfusion. This, in turn, may become colonised with anaerobic and areobic bacteria resulting in malodour and heavy exudate. Anerobic bacteria produce volatile fatty acids as a metabolic end product which cause their characteristic unpleasant smell (Grocott, 1999). This malodour can be very distressing for the patient and their family as it is a constant reminder of the situation (Kelly, 2002). It can also affect taste leading to a reduced appetite and weight loss. Heavy exudate is another problematic symptom of fungating wounds. Capillaries within the tumour are fragile and liable to haemorrhage that can be a frightening experience for the patient. Risk of bleeding also limits the amount of wound debridement that can be safely undertaken.

The management of malignant and fungating wounds can present real challenges. They may prove both physically challenging to manage and psychologically distressing for both the patient and carers. The treatment for the majority of these wounds is palliative and there is a likelihood of the wound progressing during the final stage of life. Radiotherapy and chemotherapy may be used as part of this palliative care. Malnutrition is also prevalent in cancer patients which will have a deleterious effect on the wound (Holder, 2003). A heavily exudating wound will increase protein loss further. Nutritional care in the form of nutritional supplements and pharmacological interventions will be required.

Specialist assessment

As the management of these wounds is predominately palliative, there is a need to reflect this in any assessment. Emphasis must be placed on symptom management, eg. controlling exudate leakage from dressings, rather than the condition of the wound bed itself that is likely to deteriorate. Pain, pruritis and cellulitis can also present as major problems; the patient may also present with adjacent limb lymphoedema (Grocott, 1999). A number of specialist wound assessment guides are available, including the Teler indicator (www.Teler.com). This indicator measures outcomes of patient care that are achievable using a scale of 0–5 (Grocott, 1997). Examples of patient-centred outcomes include whether a dressing is able to conform to the body, amount of leakage from the dressing and whether any additional padding needs to be applied to prevent soiling. The Teler indicator can also be applied to other wound conditions. The Wound Symptoms Self-assessment Chart (WoSSAC) (Naylor, Laverty, Mallett, 2001) is another example of a patient-focused assessment guide which also considers factors such as the effect of the wound on relationships with family and ability to socialise.

Time out

Imagine that you have just become involved in the care of a patient with a fungating wound with obvious complex needs. What referrals would you make to members of the multi-disciplinary health care team? What would be your reasoning for each of these?

Wound management

There are currently no specific dressings or formal protocols designed to cope with fungating wounds. Instead, products are chosen to cope with the main presenting problems of exudate and malodour. Suitable products for exudate include foams, alginates, hydrofibre dressings and gel sheets. Skin barriers, such as Cavilon can be useful in protecting the surrounding skin from exudate and tape damage. Non-adherent contact layers can be used as a primary dressing if the wound bed is fragile and pain is a problem.

Malodour is commonly controlled by the use of metronidazole gel (Grocott, 1999). However, in a wet wound this may be difficult to apply and may quickly become dilute. Anti-bacterial agents such as silver dressings and honey can also be used in an attempt to control malodour. Charcoal dressings also play an important role here. However, many are rendered ineffective when wet, which can be a problem in this wound type. As the wounds often occur in awkward sites or may be difficult to dress as a result of adjacent lymphoedema, getting dressings to stay in place can be difficult. A number of retention garments are available which can help dressings to stay in place without the need for lots of tape that could cause skin damage.

Pain requires accurate assessment and management as it can heighten the distress for all concerned. Grocott(1999), reports the use of topical opiates (diamorphine), local anaesthetic gels and the use of transcutaneous nerve stimulation (TENS) as being effective in the management of local wound pain and pruritis.

The risk of bleeding can be reduced by the use of non-adherent dressings and by careful wound cleansing. A number of agents are available to control bleeding. Sucralfate paste or alginate dressings are useful for slight bleeding. In the case of more severe bleeding, surgical haemostatic sponges such as Spongistan (Johnson &Johnson) can be applied (Grocott, 1999). The application of topical adrenaline has been advocated but this requires medical supervision as the resultant vasoconstriction can cause further necrosis (Naylor, 2002)

Key points

❖ Malignant wounds are areas of malignant growth and ulceration. Infiltration of malignant cells into the skin and supporting structures can result in a fungating tumour.

❖ Fungating wounds can be very distressing for the patient, their families and for any carers involved in their care

❖ The management of these wounds is predominately palliative and includes management of exudate, malodour, pain, pruritis and potential bleeding.

References

Surgical wounds

Ballard K, Baxter H (2000) *Managing acute wounds.* Essential Wound Healing Pamphlets no. 7, Johnson & Johnson, Ascot

Briggs M (1996) Surgical wound pain: a trial of two treatments. *J Wound Care* 5(10): 456–60

Briggs M (1997) Principles of closed surgical wound care. *J Wound Care* 6(6): 288–92

Chrintz H, Vibits H, Cordtz T (1989) Need for surgical wound dressings. *Br J Surgery* 76: 204–5

Desai H (1997) Ageing and wounds Part 2; healing in old age. *J Wound Care* 6(5): 237–39

Foster L, Moore P (1997) The application of a cellulose-based fibre dressing in surgical wounds. *J Wound Care* 6(10): 469–73

Harding K, Jones V (1996) *Wound Management: Good practice guidance.* J Wound Care Publication, London

Leaper D, Gottrup F (1998) Surgical wounds. In: Leaper D, Harding K, eds. *Wounds, Biology and Management.* Oxford Medical Publications, Oxford

National Institute for Clinical Excellence (2001) *Guidance on the use of debriding agents and specialist wound care clinics for difficult to heal surgical wounds, Technical Appraisal Guidance No 24.* NICE, London

Partridge C (1998) Influential factors in surgical wound repair. *J Wound Care* 7(7): 350–3

Robson M, Sampson J, Vickery C, Leaper D, Irvin T, Wainwright A, *et al* (1998) Clinical aspects of healing in specialist tissue In: Leaper D, Harding K, eds. *Wounds, Biology and Management.* Oxford Medical Publications, Oxford

Sharp C, McLaws M (2001) *Wound dressings for surgical sites* (Protocol for a Cochrane Review). In: The Cochrane library, Issue 3, Oxford: Update Software

Watret L, White R (2001) Surgical wound management: the role of dressings. *Nurs Standard* **15**(44): 59–69

White R (2001) New developments in the use of dressings on surgical wounds. *Br J Nurs* (Supplement)**10**(6): S70

Pressure ulceration

Agency for Health Care Policy and Research (1994) *Treatment of pressure ulcers: Clinical practice guidelines No. 15.* AHCPR, USA

Bennett L, Lee B (1986) Shear versus pressure as causative factors in skin blood flow occlusion *Arch Phys Med Rehab* **60**: 309–14

Bennett G, Dealey C, Posnett J (2004) The cost of pressure ulcers in the UK. *Age Ageing* **33**: 230–5

Castledine G (2003) Failure to provide adequate pressure area and personal care. Professional misconduct case studies. *Br J Nurs* **12**(8): 461

Clark M (1998) Repositioning to prevent pressure sores — what is the evidence? *Nurs Standard* **13**(3): 58–64

Clark M, Bours G, De Flour T (2003) Summary report on the prevalence of pressure ulcers. *European Pressure Ulcer Advisory Panel Review* **4**(2)

Collins F (2001) Sitting: pressure ulcer development. *Nurs Standard* **15**(22): 54–8

Cullum N, Deeks J, Sheldon T, Song F, Fletcher A (2004) Beds, mattresses and cushions for pressure sore prevention and treatment. Cochrane review. The Cochrane Library, Issue 1. John Wiley and Sons Ltd, Chichester

Department of Health (1993) *Pressure sores — a key quality indicator.* The Stationery Office, London

Department of Health (2003) *Essence of Care.* DoH, London

Dunford C (1998) Managing pressure sores. *Nurs Standard* **12**(24): 38–42

European Pressure Ulcer Advisory Panel (1998) *Pressure ulcer prevention and treatment Guidelines.* EPUAP, Oxford

Gerbhardt K, Bliss M (1994) Prevention of pressure sores in orthopaedic patients — is prolonged chair sitting detrimental? *J Tissue Viability* **4**(2): 51–4

Gray D, Cooper P, Stringfellowe S (2001) Evaluating pressure-reducing foam mattresses and electric bed frames. *Br J Nursing* (Supplement) **10**(22): S23–31

Green S, Winterberg H, Franks P, Moffatt C, McLaren S (1999) Nutritional intake in community patients with pressure ulcers. *J Wound Care* **8**(7): 325–30

Halfens R (2000) Risk assessment scales for pressure ulcers: A theoretical, methodological and clinical perspective. *Ostomy Wound Management* **46**(8): 36–44

Keogh A, Dealey C (2001) Profiling beds versus standard hospital beds: effects on pressure ulcer incidence. *J Wound Care* **10**(2): 15–19

Landis EM (1930) Micro- injections studies of capillary blood pressure in human skin. *Heart* **15**: 209–28

Lewis B (1996) Nutritional intake and the risk of pressure sore development in older patients. *J Wound Care* **7**(1): 31–5

Malone C (2000) Pressure sores in the labour ward. *RCM Midwives Journal* **3**(1): 203

Mathus-Vliegen EMH (2001) Nutritional status, nutrition and pressure ulcers. *Nutrition in Clinical Practice* **16**: 286–91

McLaren S, Green S (2001) Nutritional factors in the aetiology, development and healing of pressure ulcers. In: Morison M, ed. *The Prevention and Treatment of Pressure Ulcers*. Mosby, London

McClemont E (1984) Pressure sores. *Nurs* **2**: 21

National Institute for Clinical Excellence (2003) *Pressure ulcer prevention: Clinical Guideline 7*. NICE, London

National Institute for Clinical Excellence (2001) *Pressure ulcer risk assessment and prevention: Inherited Clinical Guideline B*. NICE, London

NHS Centre for Reviews and Dissemination (1995) Effective Health Care Bulletin. The Prevention and Treatment of Pressure Sores. NHS Centre for Reviews and Dissemination, University of York

Nixon J, McGough A (2001) Principles of patient assessment: screening for pressure ulcers and potential risk. In: Morison M, ed. *The Prevention and Treatment of Pressure Ulcers*. Mosby, London

Preston KW (1988) Positioning for comfort and pressure relief: the 30 degree alternative. *Care, Sci Practice* **6**(4): 116–19

Royal College of Nursing (2000) *Pressure ulcer risk assessment and prevention: clinical practice guidelines*. RCN, London: June

Russell L (2000) Malnutrition and pressure ulcers: nutritional assessment tools. *Br J Nurs* **9**(4): 194–204

Russell L, Reynolds T (2001) How accurate are pressure ulcer grades: an image-based survey of nurses' performance. *J Tissue Viability* **11**(2): 6775

Rycroft-Malone J, McInness E (2000) *Pressure ulcer risk assessment and prevention*. Technical Report. Royal College of Nursing, London

Strauss E, Margolis D (1996) Malnutrition in patients with pressure ulcers: morbidity, mortality and clinically practical assessments. *Adv Wound Care* **9**(5): 37–40

Tingle J (1997) Pressure sores: counting the legal cost of nursing neglect. *Br J Nurs* **6**(13): 757–8

Touche Ross (1993) *Pressure sores: A key quality indicator*. Department of Health, London

United Kingdom Central Council for Nursing, Midwifery and Health Visiting (1992) *Code of Professional Conduct*. UKCC, London

Walshe C (1995) Living with venous leg ulcer: a descriptive study of patients' experiences. *J Adv Nurs* **22**(6): 1092–100

Leg ulceration

Clinical Practice Guidelines (1998) *The Management of Patients with Venous Leg Ulcers*. The Royal College of Nursing Institute, York

Collier M (1996) Leg ulceration: a review of causes and treatment. *Nurs Standard* **10**(31): 49–51

Cornwall JV, Dore CJ, Lewis JD (1986) Leg ulcers: epidemiology and aetiology. *Br J Surgery* **73**(9): 793–6

Dale JJ, Callum MJ, Ruckley CV, Harper DR, Berry DN (1983) Chronic ulcers of the leg: a study of prevalence in a Scottish community. *Health Bull* **41**: 310–14

Davies C (2001) Use of Doppler Ultrasound in leg ulcer assessment. *Nurs Standard* **15**(44): 72–4

Franks PJ, Bosanquet N, Connolly M, Olroyd MI, Moffatt CJ, Greenhalgh RM, McCollom CN (1995) Venous ulcer healing: effect of socioeconomic factors in London. *J Epidemiol Community Health* **49**: 385–88

Laing W (1992) *Chronic Venous Diseases of the Leg*. Office of Health Economics, London

Moffat C, Dickson D (1993) The Charing Cross High Compression Four-layer Bandage System. *J Wound Care* **2**(2): 91–4

Moffatt CJ, Franks PJ, Olroyd M, Bosanquet N, Brown P, Greenhalgh RM, McCollom CN (1992) Community clinic for leg ulcers and impact on healing. *Br Med J* **305**: 1389–92

Morison M, Moffatt C (1994) *A Colour Guide to the Assessment and Management of Leg Ulcers*. 2nd edn. Mosby,

Phillips TJ (1996) Leg ulcer management. *Dermatol Nurs* **8**(5): 333–42

Rees T (2002) Use of compression therapy in venous ulceration. *Nurs Standard* **17**(6): 51–6

Vickery L, Coe N, Pearson N (1999) *The Impact of District Wide Leg Ulcer Service Developments in Somerset*. Health & Health Care Evaluation Team Directorate of Public Health & Strategy, Somerset Health Authority

Vowden K (1998) Venous leg ulcers: Part 2: Assessment. *Prof Nurse* **13**(9): 633–8

Vowden KR, Mason A, Wilkinson D, Vowden P (2000) Comparison of the healing rates and complications of three four-layer bandage regimens. *J Wound Care* **9**(6): 269–72

Diabetic foot ulceration

Bild DE *et al* (1989) Lower extremity amputation in people with diabetes: epidemiology and prevention. *Diabetes Care* **12**(1): 24–31

Brill RL, Cavanagh PR, Gibbons GW, Levin ME (1997) Treatment of Chronic Wounds. Number 7 in *Prevention of Lower Extremity Amputation in Patients with Diabetes*. Monograph made possible by an educational grant from Curative Health Services, Inc. Online at: http://www.curative.com

Curley MA, Quigley SM, Lin M (2003) Pressure ulcers in pediatric intensive care: incidence and associated factors. *Pediatr Crit Care Med* **4**(3): 383–4

Currie CJ *et al* (1997) NHS Acute Sector Expenditure for Diabetes: The present, future and excess in-patient cost of care. *Diabetic Med* **14**: 686–92

Foster A (2000) *Essential Wound Healing Part 9: Diabetic Foot Ulceration*. Emap Healthcare, London

Scottish Intercollegiate Guidelines Network (2001) *Guideline 55, Section 7: Management of Diabetic Foot Disease*. SIGN, Edinburgh

King KM (2003) Diabetes: classification and strategies for integrated care. *Br J Nurs* **12**(20): 1204–10

Larsen K, Fabrin J, Holstein PE (2001) Incidence and management of ulcers in diabetic Charcot feet. *J Wound Care* **10**(8): 323–8

Young MJ *et al* (1994) The prediction of diabetic neuropathic foot ulceration using vibration

Burns

Atkinson A (1998) Nursing burn wounds on general wards. *Nurs Standard* **12**(41): 58–67

Dearden C, Donnell J, Dunlop M, Higgins M, Tieney E (2001) Traumatic wounds: The management of superficial and partial thickness burns. *Nurs Times Plus* **97**(48): 53–5

European Tissue Repair Society (1999) Guidelines for the outpatient treatment of 1st and 2nd degree burns. In: Benbow, Burg, Martinez, Erikson *et al*, eds. *Guidelines for the Outpatient Treatment of Chronic Wounds and Burns*. Blackwell Science, Berlin

Flanagan M, Graham J (2001) Should burn blisters be left intact or debrided? *J Wound Care* **10**(1): 41–4

Fowler A, Burns (1999) In: Miller M, Glover D, eds. *Wound Management, Theory and Practice*. NT books, London

Regojo P (2003) Burn care basics. *Nursing* **33**(3): 50–5

Richard R (1998) Assessment and diagnosis of burn wounds. *Adv Wound Care* **12**(9): 468–71

Taylor K (2001) Burns and scalds in children. *Nurs Standard* **16**(11): 45–51

Tortora G, Grabowski S (2000) *Principles of Anatomy and Physiology*. 9th edn. Wiley and Sons, New York

Wardrope J, Edhouse J (1998) *The Management of Wounds and Burns*. 2nd edn. Oxford University Press, Oxford

Malignant and fungating wounds

Adderley U, Smith R (2002) *Topical agents and dressings for fungating wounds (Protocol for a Cochrane Review)*. In: The Cochrane Library, Issue 3, Oxford, Update software

Akguner M, Barutcu A, Yilmaz M, Karatas O, Vayvada H (1998) Marjolin's ulcer and chronic burn scarring. *J Wound Care* **7**(3): 121–2

Grocott P (1997) Evaluation of a tool used to assess the management of fungating wounds. *J Wound Care* **6**(9): 421–4

Grocott P (1999) The management of fungating wounds. *J Wound Care* **8**(5): 232–4

Haisfield-Wolfe M, Rund C (1997) Malignant cutaneous wounds: a management protocol. *Ostomy Wound Management* **43**(1): 56–66

Holder H (2003) Nursing management of nutrition in cancer and palliative care. *Br J Nurs* **12**(11): 667–74

Kelly N (2002) Malodourous wounds: a review of current literature. *Prof Nurse* **17**(5): 323–6

Naylor W (2002) Part 1. Symptom control in the management of fungating wounds. Online at: www.World wide wounds.com

Naylor W, Laverty D, Mallett (2001) *The Royal Marsden Hospital Handbook of Wound Management in Cancer Care*. Blackwell Science,

Chapter 5

Advanced, specialist and alternative therapies

This chapter will introduce you to a number of advanced and alternative wound care therapies that are becoming increasingly more available. Some of these therapies are traditional therapies with histories of usage spanning hundreds if not thousands of years. Other therapies are new developments using complex tissue engineering that works at a cellular level or mechanical devices that again can stimulate wound healing. A case study illustrating the use of a number of advances/alternative therapies is included in *Appendix 4*.

Vacuum-assisted wound closure

Definition

Vacuum-assisted wound closure is a method of wound management that relies on the application of a uniform negative pressure to the base of the wound. It is also referred to as topical negative pressure (Banwell and Toet, 2003). This negative pressure is achieved by applying a reticulated foam dressing and drainage tube to the wound. This is then occluded with a drape and attached to a vacuum pump (VAC, KCI Medical). When the negative pressure is applied the foam collapses and the resultant forces are transmitted to all wound surfaces in contact with the foam dressing. *Figures 5.1* and *5.2* illustrate a VAC system and a wound pre and post VAC therapy.

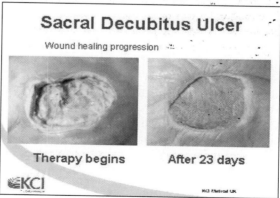

Figure 5.1: Vac therapy pump

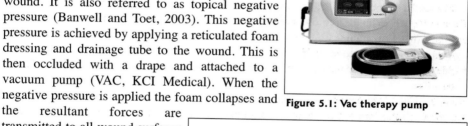

Figure 5.2: Wound pre and post VAC therapy

Effects on wound bed

Initially, vacuum-assisted wound closure works by removing excess interstitial fluid. This fluid can collect and impede the delivery of oxygen and nutrients to the wound bed as it compromises the microcirculation and lymphatics (Argenta and Morykwas, 1997). Once this is achieved, there is an increased vascularity of the wound bed that will result in the production of healthy granulation tissue at an early stage. Other advantages of negative pressure include the removal of bacteria and inhibiting factors (proteolytic enzymes and matrix metalloproteinases) which are found in chronic wound fluid and disrupt healing. This method of wound healing relies on an air-tight seal — there is no leakage of fluid or odour from the dressing. This method can be advantageous in difficult to handle, wet wounds.

Suitability

Although the use of vacuum-assisted wound closure is becoming widespread, both within the hospital and community setting, it remains a specialist product and should not be applied to a patient without appropriate supervision and training. It is important to ensure that a sufficient number of staff are trained so that all dressings can be undertaken and any potential problems dealt with competently throughout the treatment episode. A good application technique is required in order to avoid unnecessary skin damage and to prevent leaks within the system which will disable the machine. The pump also needs to be set up safely. The optimum pressure setting is 125mmHg but this may vary according to the wound and patient conditions. This pressure is applied on a continuous setting initially. Intermittent therapy using a seven-minute cycle (five minutes on and two minutes off) has also been found to be beneficial in stimulating healing and is recommended for a number of wound types.

To ensure that optimum benefit is gained from this therapy, wound bed preparation is important. Granulation tissue cannot be generated in the presence of necrotic tissue so steps to remove this may need to be taken beforehand (ie. sharp or surgical debridement). Wounds require careful monitoring and dressings are usually changed every forty-eight hours. To prevent trauma to the wound bed and surrounding skin, agents such as silicone skin protectors, thin hydrocolloids and silicone contact layers may be used. This therapy is not usually continued to the end point of healing but is discontinued when the wound can be easily managed using conventional products or covered with a skin graft.

There are an increasing body of case studies and research studies that indicate the growing number of areas where vacuum-assisted wound closure can be successfully used. It is now widely used in surgical wounds, such as: wound dehiscence, infected sternotomy wounds, traumatic soft tissue injuries, delayed wound closure and in skin flap and graft repairs of skin defects including degloving injuries (Morykwas and Argenta, 1997; Harlan, 2002; Scherer *et al*, 2002; Clare *et al*, 2002). A recent development has been its use in the treatment of open abdomens using a specialist dressing to protect the exposed organs and also in enteric fistulas (Banwell and Teot, 2003). The use of negative pressure is well documented in the treatment of chronic wounds, such as leg ulcers and pressure ulcers and, more recently, diabetic ulcers.

A small portable pump is available which is suitable for community use. A number of foam types and dressing options are also available.

Contraindications and precautions

These currently include malignancy due to the risk of dispersing diseased cells, untreated osteomyelitis, exposed blood vessels and organs, non-enteric and unexplored fistulas and where there is dry necrotic tissue present. There are also a number of precautions, including active bleeding and patients on anti-coagulant therapy (KCI, 2003).

> **Time out**
>
> What information would you want to know if you were a patient with a complex wound and vacuum-assisted wound drainage had been recommended. Do you currently have sufficient knowledge and understanding to answer questions and to explain its main features?

Cost-effectiveness

The rental or purchase cost of the machine together with the purchase cost of the dressings and disposables is high (approximately £60 a day). However, this is offset by the anticipated decrease in healing time. A major disadvantage of this system is that the dressings are not available on drug tariff which may restrict its use, particularly in the community.

Key points

❖ Vacuum-assisted wound closure is a method of wound closure that relies on the application of a uniform negative pressure to the base of the wound.

❖ The main action of this therapy is the removal of excess interstitial fluid. This leads to an increased vascularity of the wound bed that will result in the production of healthy granulation tissue at an early stage.

❖ The use of vacuum-assisted wound closure is becoming widespread both within the hospital and community setting and on a wide variety of wound conditions. However, it remains a specialist product and should not be applied to a patient without appropriate supervision and training.

Larval (maggot) therapy

There have been numerous reports spanning many hundreds of years of the beneficial effects of maggots in wounds. In most cases the maggots had accidentally entered the wound (myiasis), particularly in battle ground situations. The accidental finding of maggots in wounds is not an unusual event even today, and these experiences are rarely forgotten.

The practice of introducing maggots in wounds as a debridement agent became common during the 1930s, especially in America. Its popularity decreased during the 1940s with the advent of antibiotics. The use of maggots was revived in the 1980s and became increasingly more popular in the 1990s (Thomas *et al*, 1999).

Sterile maggots are now produced in a number of countries including the UK, Israel, Germany, Hungary and the Ukraine.

The maggot used for biosurgery is the greenbottle fly, *Lucilia sericata*. It is the fly of choice as the enzymes produced only dissolve dead tissue in humans and the maggots are therefore unable to digest viable tissue. The epidermis which is avascular, may be digested if not protected.

Mode of action

Maggots are effective in removing necrotic tissue and combating infection, there is also evidence to suggest that their presence in a wound can stimulate wound healing.

Larvae secrete a powerful mix of proteolytic enzymes which dissolve the wound debris and turn it into a form of nutritious soup: contrary to popular belief, the larvae drink rather than eat the dead tissue. These secretions can cause the wound exudate to become discoloured to a dark red colour. This should be explained to the staff and patient in order to avoid concern. The anti-microbial acitivity of maggots is not confined to the secretions alone. Bacteria ingested by the larvae are destroyed as they pass through their gut (Robinson and Norwood, 1933). The secretions will also reduce the wound pH due to the production of ammonia. This acidic environment is hostile to bacteria. Studies have shown maggots to be effective against Gram positive bacteria such as *Staphylococcus* and *Streptococcus* including MRSA (Thomas *et al*, 1999). The authors suggest that it is likely that the various functions that the maggots perform work synergistically within the wound.

Indications for use

The main use for larval therapy has been in the treatment of necrotic and sloughy wounds, such as pressure and leg ulcers. They have also been used for osteomyelitis, malignant wounds, necrotising fasciitis, diabetic foot ulcers, burns and to prepare sites for grafting (see case study). The contraindications for their use include fistulas, or wounds that might connect to vital organs. Unfortunately, larvae therapy is often used as a last resort and will not be effective in patients where the main problem is a lack of blood supply to the limb. Patients may be aware of the larvae and may complain of a mild 'picking' sensation, although an increase in pain in patients with ischaemic limbs has been reported (Thomas *et al*, 2001; Wayman *et al*, 1999). *Figure 5.3* illustrates larvae within a wound.

> ### Time out
>
> How would you feel if you were asked to apply larvae to one of your patients? If you find that you are reluctant to do this consider the reasons why. How could you overcome these?

Larvae life cycle

The eggs are sterilised to ensure that the outer surface is free of bacteria. Once hatched, the larvae measure 1–2mm in length and will grow rapidly over the next three to five days to reach 8mm in length. The transition of larvae to fly usually takes seven to ten days according to temperature. The maximum time that the larvae are left on the wound is three days in order to avoid this transition.

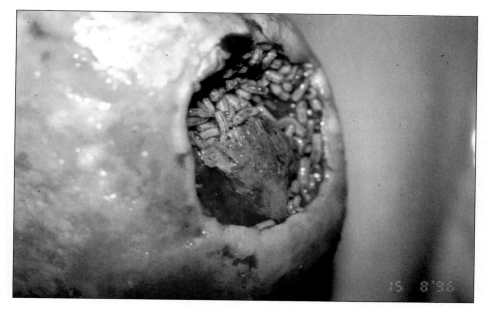

Figure 5.3: Larval therapy, courtesy of Steve Thomas

Cost-effectiveness

The unit cost of larvae is quite high and more than one tube may be required. Thomas *et al* (2001) suggests that in the long term it may be more cost-effective to use a larger number of maggots in a single application than extended treatments with small numbers of maggots. The current situation is that larval therapy has recently been added to the drug tariff which means that many community patients will now be eligible for this treatment. Wayman *et al* (1999), looked at the cost-effectiveness of larvae versus hydrogel in the debridement of leg ulcers which showed a cost comparison of £79 for larvae and £136 for the control group. Nursing time was significantly greater for the control group which required daily dressings.

Application

This is a specialist technique and training in their application is required. The priority is to protect the surrounding skin from the secretions which is usually achieved by using a hydrocolloid dressing as a template. It is necessary to ensure the survival of the larvae by allowing them to breathe while also keeping them on the wound; a nylon mesh dressing is applied over the larvae and secured onto the hydrocolloid. For foot or digit wounds, mesh bags are supplied to go over the limb. The larvae are removed on the third day and incinerated. Their survival rate will vary and will be influenced by the amount of debris and oxygen available. Hydrogels containing glycol have been shown to be harmful to the larvae (Thomas *et al*, 1998). Depending on the condition of the wound, a fresh batch of larvae or a conventional dressing may be applied as required (Thomas *et al*, 1998).

Larvae are now available in a soft polyvinylkalcohol bag which can be applied to the wound. This results in easier application and removal and means that they are invisible to patient and staff which may help overcome the 'yuk' factor (Thomas *et al*, 2001).

Key points

❖ Maggots are effective in removing necrotic tissue and combating infection. There is also evidence to suggest that their presence in a wound can stimulate wound healing.

❖ The main use for larval therapy has been in the treatment of necrotic and sloughy wounds, such as pressure and leg ulcers.

❖ Larval therapy is a specialist technique and training in their application is required. The priority is to protect the surrounding skin from the secretions, which is usually achieved by using a hydrocolloid dressing as a template.

Honey

Honey has been used in wound healing for many centuries. Jones (2001) states that evidence for the use of medicinal honey has been found in Asian, Chinese and Egyptian texts dating back over 2000 years and that there are many biblical references to it. Honey's uses were not limited to wound healing and included contraception, laxative, diuretic, eye conditions, pneumonia and snake bites, to name but a few.

Mode of action

Similar to larval therapy, the use of honey became all but forgotten with the advent of antibiotics and modern dressings. In recent years there has been a renewed interest in honey as a wound healing agent, and it has received local and national publicity and generated a lot of public interest (Lord, 2000). Much of this interest has revolved around Leptospermum honeys from Australia and New Zealand, often referred to as Manuka honeys. There is a growing body of scientific evidence and case studies which indicates the efficacy of certain honeys in stimulating wound healing (Molan, 1999). These wound healing properties are shown in *Table 5.1*. Leptospermum honeys have a high antibacterial component from nectar, making it a good choice for wound healing. Another advantage is that the antiseptic properties of honey are not harmful to cells (Cooper and Molan, 1999). As honey can contain spores of clostridia, honey for wound management should be sterilised using Gamma-irradiation.

Honey has been successfully used for a number of different wound types including burns (Subrahmanyam, 1998), superficial wounds (Harris, 1994) and infected and chronic wounds including leg ulcers (Dunford *et al*, 2000; Kingsley 2001). However, there remains a lack of randomised controlled trials to support fully honey's role in wound healing (Moore *et al*, 2001). Although there is only a theoretical risk of honey disturbing blood glucose levels, diabetic patients should be regularly monitored while using honey products.

Table 5.1: Wound healing properties of honey

Antibacterial activity

- Inhibits a wide range of Gram-negative and positive bacteria and fungi
- Powerful deodoriser

Anti-inflammatory properties

- Reduction of oedema
- Reduction of pain

Stimulation of wound healing

- Stimulates debridement and phagocytosis
- Stimulates angiogenesis (formation of granulation tissue)
- Cell proliferation
- Collagen synthesis
- Re-epithelialization

Disadvantages

Can be difficult to apply and keep in place as it liquifies with higher temperatures

Not currently available on Drug Tariff

Some patients experience a slight pulling and stinging sensation

adapted from Cooper, 2000

Application of honey

The amount of honey required and frequency of dressing change will depend on the amount of exudate present and the size of the wound. The general rule is that 20mls of honey should be sufficient for a 10cm x 10cm dressing. It has been recommended that dressings are changed daily and more frequently if the wound is heavily exudating to prevent the honey becoming too dilute (Molan and Betts, 2000). This is not realistic within many healthcare settings. Removal of the honey does not usually present a problem and the application of warm water will quickly counteract any adherence. The use of honey can cause skin staining but this is easily removed on gentle washing.

A range of honey products, including impregnated dressings, alginates, and honey gels have recently been added to the Drug Tariff.

Key points

❖ There has been a renewed interest in honey as a wound healing agent, particularly in the use of honeys from Australia and New Zealand that are often referred to as Manuka honeys.

❖ It is proving successful as a wound healing agent due to its antibacterial, anti-inflammatory and cell stimulating properties.

❖ There remains a lack of randomised controlled studies to fully support honey's role in wound healing.

Tissue engineering

Definition

The potential for most human tissue to repair or regenerate ensures that the majority of wounds, particularly minor ones, will heal uneventfully given reasonable care. Nevertheless, it should never be overlooked that wound healing is, at the least, a complex interdependent cellular and molecular process (Gope, 2002). The healthy wound bed is a highly regulated environment rather like a well run building site in a brownfield area.

Where the wound area is extensive or the patient has concurrent chronic illness, the wound healing process may be impaired as a result of a biochemical or cellular imbalance. In an environment where there are multiple and interrelated chemical cascades occurring which simultaneously stimulate or inhibit activity, it is not hard to imagine the microcosmic chaos caused if certain essential components are missing or a process fails to halt when required to do so. In diabetes, for example, there may be a decreased ability by the body to synthesise normal matrix proteins (Mulder, 1999). Wound healing may become static despite the absence of infection and the use of appropriate wound dressings.

In recent years, these and similar problems, have motivated researchers to look more closely at the microbiological processes of wound healing. This work has led to the development of materials, derived from or resembling human tissue and its extra-cellular components, that can be applied to wounds to augment healing. This new technology is called tissue engineering and has been defined as:

> ... the development of new materials or devices capable of specific interactions with biological tissues. In wound care, these materials may be based entirely on naturally occurring tissues and cells.
>
> Sefton and Woodhouse, 1998

Some of the products available may be designed to activate one particular process, eg. angiogenesis (the development of new blood vessels) or they may be extremely complex materials, such as bilayered human skin equivalents. These contain both the cellular and acellular features of normal skin plus other chemotaxic and proliferating agents, such as growth factors and matrix proteins.

Autologous grafts

Human skin grafting has been used for centuries (Eaglstein and Falanga, 1998). The most successful usage was, until recently, autogenic (derived from the individual on which it was used). This was because of the problems of rejection and the risk of disease transmission. However, sufficient healthy skin is not always available, this is especially the case in patients with large burns where intact skin may be limited. In addition, the harvesting of an individual's own skin creates further wounds at a time when they are already immunologically stressed. The additional pain and risk of infection and scarring may well further compromise the healing process.

Cultured autologous keratinocytes

To address this problem considerable work was done to find ways to increase the supply of autologous tissue. One solution is to culture the patient's own epithelial cells taken from a small skin biopsy (Johnson, 2000). Although the risk of rejection is avoided, the main drawback to this method is that the process is time-consuming, with a three- to four-week delay, and requires the underpinning technology to produce the cells. What practitioners needed was a quicker solution.

Human allografts

The need for an off-the-shelf product led to the development of allografts (prepared from tissue taken from one individual for use on another) that would not be so easily rejected. These products, derived from processed human cadaver skin are cryogenically stored when prepared and reconstituted prior to use. During manufacture, those components that would stimulate an autologous response are removed to produce an immunologically inert product (Mulder, 1999).

Although the problem of rejection and ready availability has been solved, some anxiety about disease transmission remains. Donor screening for viruses, especially those of hepatitis and HIV, as well as bacterial and fungal infections is required. Despite the most rigorous screening it is possible for skin from HIV infected donors who are seronegative to be passed as suitable for use (Eaglstein and Falanga, 1998).

Cultured allogenic keratinocytes

Another development was the production of cultured allogous cells. Instead of cadaveric skin, human epithelial cells, taken from newly circumcised foreskins are used. These cells which become immunologically inert during culture are manufactured in large quantities and produced in sheets. These are then transposed onto gauze and cryopreserved ready for use. A disadvantage is that epithelial cells are fragile and have no dermis, which may limit their cosmetic effect (Eaglstein and Falanga, 1998).

Human dermal replacement

An improved solution was to create an immunologically inert, but metabolically active dermal layer using fibroblasts from neonatal foreskins rather than cadaveric skin. This material is complete with normal dermal matrix proteins and cytokines. This surface stimulates the production of the patients own cells but, if required, spilt skin grafts can also be applied on top. The fibroblasts are cultured and grown on a bioabsorbable mesh. As they proliferate, dermal collagen and growth factors are produced. The risk of infection does remain and to avoid this, maternal blood is screened for exposure to infectious diseases as part of the production process.

Human skin equivalent

The greatest leap forward so far has been the development of bi-layered products which contain both a dermal and an epidermal layer. This solves many of the problems experienced with earlier products but there are limitations. Although it is designed to look and feel like ordinary skin (Johnson, 2000), it does not contain immune cells or melanocytes. There are also no skin structures such as sweat glands, hair follicles or blood vessels. It is therefore translucent and may not match the patient's own skin tones. Nevertheless, much work continues to be done and the objective of custom-controlled skin equivalent is said to be achievable (Johnson, 2000).

Time out

The products mentioned so far are based on skin. Take a few moments to compare the functions of the skin (*p.1*) with the characteristics of an ideal dressing (*p.30–35*). What factors are similar and what are different? Can tissue engineering products be classed as dressings?

Growth factors and proteolytic enzyme inhibitors

The products listed so far were designed for use on acute wounds, but as the understanding of the physiology of wound healing developed, there was an increased hope that the management of chronic wounds could also be improved. Manufacturers responded by marketing products containing specific chemical components, thought to be missing in slow to heal wounds. One large group of this type of product are the growth factors. Growth factors are produced within the normal healing wound and each one is responsible for stimulating proliferation of respondent cells and/or other related activities. For example, epidermal growth factor stimulates the production of epithelial cells whereas fibroblast growth factor, among other functions, will stimulate angiogenesis. In poorly healing wounds, certain growth factors may be absent or reduced in supply.

Other products have been designed not to stimulate but to inhibit activity thought to be harmful to the healing wound. Proteases are enzymes which degrade collagen and break down other unwanted materials that need to be cleared from the healing wound. Sometimes the process gets out of control and newly synthesised collagen is destroyed (Casey, 2002). Protease inhibitors are designed to prevent undesired tissue breakdown. The developments so far described are not exhaustive. There are many others and new ones are coming onto the market everyday.

Dressings or treatments?

Wound dressings have come a long way from the time when they were made from the cotton waste off the factory floor. At that time they did little more than cover the wound and absorb exudate. As knowledge about wound healing increased, modern wound dressings were developed to create and promote the healing environment. Terms such as occlusive, hydrophyllic and semi-permeable were used as descriptors of these products. Tissue engineering appears to add another dimension to the management of wound healing.

Time out

Consider the features of an ideal dressing (*p. 30*). How do these new products differ?

The purpose of tissue engineered products is to attempt to correct abnormalities in the healing cascade, similar to some antibacterial products, but most incorporate few, if any, of the other features of an ideal dressing. Only a handful of dressings were cited by Harding *et al* (2002) as actively promoting, as well as assisting, healing. Tissue engineered products are perhaps best regarded as wound treatments rather than wound dressings.

Indications for use

Tissue engineering is undoubtedly the way forward. Currently, although some products have had good results others have proved as yet disappointing. Some products are very expensive. Most are not available on prescription and although it can be argued that if they worked they would be cost effective, if they fail for whatever reason, both the practitioner and patient are left frustrated and disillusioned.

One of the main difficulties is that it is impossible for the average practitioner to know what, if anything, is lacking at a biochemical level, in the wound they are caring for. Without a simple test to identify any deficiencies, selecting the appropriate product is all too much of a 'hit and miss' affair. Also, other additional physiological factors may still delay the healing process. Practitioners need help from manufacturers and researchers to overcome these practical problems to use these products more effectively.

Patient scenario seven.

Would any of the advanced/alternative wound management products discussed in this chapter be suitable for the treatment of Mr Skelton's pressure ulcer and, if so, why? (see *Figure 2.7*).

Treatment options:

Reasoning:

Key points

❖ Tissue engineering and has been defined as 'the development of new materials or devices capable of specific interactions with biological tissues. In wound care, these materials may be based entirely on naturally occurring tissues and cells' (Sefton and Woodhouse, 1998).

❖ These products should be classed as wound treatments rather than wound dressings.

❖ Although they are being developed and improved all the time, currently there is no simple test which can tell the practitioner what, if anything, is missing from the wound bed.

References

Vacuum-assisted wound closure

Argenta LC, Morykwas MJ (1997) Vacuum-assisted closure: a new method for wound control and treatment: Clinical experiences. *Ann Plastic Surgery* **38**(6): 563–76

Banwell P, Toet L (2003) Topical negative pressure (TNP): the evolution of a novel wound therapy. *J Wound Care* **12**(1): 22–8

Clare MP, Fitzgibbons TC, McMullen ST, Stice RC, Hayes DR, Henkel L (2002) Experience with the vacuum-assisted closure negative pressure technique in the treatment of non-healing diabetic and dysvascular wounds. *Foot Ankle International* **23**(10): 896–901

Harlan JW (2002) Treatment of open sternal wounds with the vacuum-assisted system: a safe, reliable method. *Plastic Reconstructive Surgery* **109**(2): 710–12

KCI (2003) *VAC Therapy, Clinical Guidelines*. KCI Medical Ltd, Witney

Morykwas MJ, Argenta LC (1997) Vacuum-assisted wound closure: A new method for wound control and treatment: Clinical experience. *Ann Plastic Surg* **38**(6): 553–62

Scherer LA, Shiver S, Chang M, Meredith JW, Owings JT (2002) The vacuum-assisted closure device. A method of securing skin grafts and improving graft survival. *Arch Surg* **137**(8): 930–4

Larval therapy

Robinson W, Norwood VH (1933) The role of surgical maggots in the disinfection of osteomyelitis and other infected wounds. *J Bone Joint Surg* **15**: 409–12

Thomas S, Andrews , Jones M (1998) The use of larval therapy in wound management. *J Wound Care* **7**(10): 521–4

Thomas S, Andrews, Hay, Bourgoise (1999) The anti-microbial maggot secretions: results of a preliminary study. *J Tissue Viability* **9**(4): 127–31

Thomas S, Jones M, Wynn K, Fowler T (2001) The current status of maggot therapy in wound healing. *Br J Nurs* (Supplement) **10**(22): S5-S 12

Wayman J, Nirojogi, Walker, Sowinski (1999) The cost effectiveness of larval therapy in venous ulcers. *J Tissue Viability* **10**(3): 91–4

Honey

Cooper R, Molan P (1999) The use of honey as an antiseptic in managing *Pseudomonas* infection. *J Wound Care* **8**(4): 161–4

Cooper R (2000) How does honey heal wounds? In: Munn, Jones M, eds. *Honey and Healing*. IBRA, Cardiff

Dunford C, Cooper R, Molan P, White R (2000) The use of honey in wound management. *Nurs Standard* **15**(11): 63–8

Harris S (1994) Honey for the treatment of superficial wounds: a case report and review. *Primary Intention* **2**(4): 18–23

Jones R (2001) Honey and healing through the ages. In: Munn , Jones M, eds. *Honey and healing*. IBRA, Cardiff

Kingsley A (2001) The use of honey in the treatment of infected wounds: case studies. *Br J Nurs* (suppl) **10**(22): S13–S20

Lord A (2000) Sweet healing. *New Scientist* **168**(2259): 32–5

Molan P (1999) The role of honey in the management of wounds. *J Wound Care* **8**(8): 415–18

Molan P (1999) Why honey is effective as a medicine.1. Its use in modern medicine. *Bee World* **80**(2): 80–92

Molan P, Betts J (2000) Using honey dressings: the practical considerations. *Nurs Times* **96**(49): 36–7

Moore O, Smith L, Campbell F, Seers K, McQuay H, Moore A (2001) Systematic review of the use of honey as a wound dressing. *Complementary and Alternative Medicine* 1: 2 (Online at: www.biomedcentral.com)

Subrahmanyam M (1998) A prospective randomised clinical and histological study of superficial burn wound healing with honey and silver sulphadiazine. *Burns* **24**(2): 157–61

Tissue engineering

Casey G (2002) Wound repair: Advanced dressing materials. *Nurs Standard* **17**(4): 49

Eaglstein WH, Falanga V (1998) *Tissue engineering and the use of Apligraf, a human skin equivalent*. Cutis Chatham 62 Iss 1S 1-8

Gope R (2002) The effect of epidermal growth factor and platelet derived growth factors on wound healing process. *Indian J Med Res* **6**: 201

Harding KG, Morris HL, Patel GK (2002) Healing chronic wounds. *Br Med J* **324**(730):160

Johnson PC (2000) The role of tissue engineering. *Adv Skin Wound Care* **1**(3) (suppl 2): 12–14

Mulder GT (1999) The role of tissue engineering in wound care. *J Wound Care* **8**(1): 21–4

Sefton MV, Woodhouse KA (1998) Tissue engineering. *J Cutaneous Med Surg* **3** (suppl 1): 18–23

Chapter 6

The role of tissue viability within modern health care

Clinical governance

Since its foundation in 1948, the National Health Service has seen a number of major structural and organisational changes over the years. The *NHS Plan*, published in July 2000, set out the Labour Government's intention to push forward a radical programme of modernisation directed at improving the care provided. As part of this initiative a number of taskforces were established to concentrate on specific issues. One of these taskforces centred on the quality of the care provided to ensure that care delivery was evidence-based and consistent with best practice.

This approach to care delivery is called clinical governance (first outlined in the White Paper of 1997, *The New NHS, Modern and Dependable*). It has now been adopted as a framework for ensuring that NHS organisations and care providers are accountable. This accountability exists not only at a corporate but also at an individual level, and extends beyond the standard of care currently provided to include the future. Each NHS worker is obligated to strive continually for improvement, thus creating an environment where clinical excellence can flourish.

Clinical governance has implications for tissue viability practitioners, who must ensure that the care they provide has a clear rationale. They are also required to keep up-to-date with new developments within the field.

The National Service Frameworks (NSFs)

The *NHS Plan* (2000) also re-emphasised the role of the national service frameworks. These frameworks, launched as a rolling programme in 1998, cover a range of conditions or groups or areas of care, which the government believed, required specific attention. Tissue viability issues are highlighted in some of these frameworks. In *The National Service Framework for Older People* (2001), tissue viability is one of the set of standardised domains of patient assessment and pressure ulcer risk assessment is particularly highlighted. Conditions, such as leg ulcers and peripheral vascular disease, are also mentioned.

The single assessment process and interprofessional working

One particular initiative to come from *The National Service Framework for Older People* is the single assessment process. This is designed to prevent duplication and foster closer co-operation between those professionals involved in one patient's care. This ensures that assessments are carried out by the professional with the most appropriate skills. Gaps can be quickly identified and an improved recognition of each individual contribution promoted. The Government believes that closer interprofessional working will lead to more effective care provision which will benefit the patient (Kenny, 2002).

Tissue viability is one area where a multidisciplinary approach to care is particularly useful. The assessment and interventions involved in the prevention of pressure ulcers, for example, may include physiotherapists, dieticians and occupational therapists as well as doctors and nurses; whereas close co-operation between podiatrists and tissue viability practitioners may well improve care for the patient with a diabetic foot ulcer.

The changing nursing role

Together with greater accountability and closer co-operation with other professional groups, the role of the nurse is changing in other ways too. Nurses are moving into areas that were formerly the exclusive preserve of others. The development of nurse consultant posts and nurse prescribing has enhanced nursing status. The *NHS Plan* (2000) sets out the Government's intention that suitably qualified and trained nurses should be empowered to admit and discharge patients, order investigations and run clinics. Nurse-led tissue viability and leg ulcer clinics are now commonplace and nurses are more likely to advise doctors on dressing usage than the reverse. Tissue viability is, indeed, an area where a considerable amount of professional autonomy is possible.

Patient advocacy and empowerment

If nurses are being challenged within the health service to improve standards of care, they are also being challenged by patients themselves. The *NHS Plan* requires care providers to put patients at the centre of their activities and formally to provide them with a say in all aspects of their care. Two of the developments designed to achieve this outcome has been the Patients Advice and Liaison Service (PALS) and patient forums. Information is more readily available nowadays and the internet and other sources of advice and knowledge are increasingly being accessed by patients.

Patient choice is a central precept of modern health care, but the ability to make informed choice depends on the patient being properly equipped to make those choices. Professionals can no longer hide behind the 'doctor (or nurse) knows best' scenario. We are obligated to educate and inform our patients and encourage them to take control of their lives and their health problems. The tissue viability practitioner teaching a paraplegic man to check his skin for pressure damage with a hand-held mirror is an example of this.

Litigation

As a society we are becoming more litigious and untoward occurrences such as an avoidable pressure ulcer, besides being a source of pain and anxiety for the patient and stress for staff, can also cost the NHS a great deal of money that would otherwise go to patient care. We owe our patients a duty of care and to provide that care at the required standard. The importance of careful assessment, evidence-based planning, documented intervention and timely evaluation will reduce the risk of litigation. Even when things do go wrong, if it can be demonstrated that the appropriate care was planned and provided at the appropriate level, then the practitioner has met their obligation and can do no more.

Policies and guidelines

If increased autonomy and independence in practice has provided greater intellectual rewards and job satisfaction for practitioners, it has also meant increased responsibility. This can be extremely daunting for the newly qualified professional. Knowledge may be available in books, but experience can only be acquired. Guidelines, policies, care pathways and other tools provide a structured framework that the practitioner can work safely within. They set out the standard of care expected and although they may not hold all the answers, they provide a solid basis for practice. Some documents may be in-house, developed locally, or be available nationally. The *Clinical Practice Guidelines for the Management of Patients with Venous Leg Ulcers* (1998) and those for pressure ulcer prevention (2003) are national examples pertinent to tissue viability practitioners.

Reflection

Throughout professional life we never stop learning and we have to develop effective ways to process new information quickly in order to update continuously and consolidate our practice. All professional experiences, good or bad, can be put to positive use in that they provide us with a learning opportunity. Reflection is a very useful tool for all practitioners, at whatever level, in helping to improve performance. By setting aside time to look at events in a structured way, to consider the positive and negative elements and to consider what might have been done to achieve an improved outcome will prepare the practitioner mentally for the same or similar events occurring in the future.

Audit and benchmarking

Benchmarking is another useful tool to enable individual practitioners or teams to see how well they are doing. Initially developed in eight aspects of care, the level of care provided is measured against a set of given standards so that any shortcomings can be identified. The tool facilitates an exploration as to why the standard might not have been met and assists in the identification of ways in which best practice can be achieved. Good practice is to be shared among practitioners and poor practice improved.

Benchmarking on the prevention of pressure ulcers was outlined in the *Essence of Care* (DoH, 2003).

Competing agendas

As allocators of public resources, healthcare practitioners have an obligation to use them wisely. Dilemmas as to whether provision for patient 'A' may deprive patient 'B' and whether provision should be based on equity or equality are often a source of great anxiety for individual practitioners. Many dressings and treatments used in the management of wounds are expensive, as are specialised pressure-reducing and relieving mattresses. Fair allocation often means that tough decisions have to be made.

Whereas previously there may have been a division between care providers and budget holders, practitioners increasingly occupy both roles. This makes the rationing aspect of health care more explicit and exposes the ethical dimension within current practice. Resources are finite, but the practitioner has a duty to ensure that the best possible value for money is obtained.

References

Clinical Practice Guidelines (1998) *The Management of Patients with Venous Leg Ulcers*. The Royal College of Nursing Institute, York

Department of Health (1997) *The New NHS, Modern Dependable*. DoH, London

Department of Health (2000) *The NHS Plan: A Plan for Investment: A Plan for Reform*. DoH, London

Department of Health (2001) *National Service Framework for Older People*. DoH, London

Department of Health (2003) *Patient Focused Benchmarks for Healthcare Practitioners*. CNO Publications, London

Department of Health (2002) Essence of Care. DoH, London

Kenny G (2002) Interprofessional working: opportunities and challenges. *Nurs Standard* **17**(6): 33–5

Royal College of Nursing (2000) *Pressure ulcer risk assessment and prevention: clinical practice guidelines*. RCN, London

Summative quiz

1. Mrs Sinclair is eighty-three years old and is admitted to your ward with emphysema which is making her very breathless and distressed. To aid her breathing she sits out in a chair but she still finds it difficult to eat and talk. You notice a reddened area on her sacrum with epidermal loss.

   What are the priorities in her care?
   a) Contact the tissue viability nurse ☐
   b) Undertake a thorough wound assessment including pressure
      ulcer grading ☐
   c) Educate Mrs Sinclair and her family on the effects of pressure
   d) Immediately remove her from the chair so that no further pressure
      can be applied ☐
   e) Refer to local policies and guidelines as to what to do ☐
   f) Sit Mrs Sinclair on a pillow to relieve pressure ☐

2. You are asked to grade the pressure ulcer as part of your wound assessment. What grade from the EPUAP grading scale would be appropriate for this ulcer?

3. What questions should you ask Mrs Sinclair to determine if her nutritional status is adding to her risk of pressure ulceration?

4. You are present when a colleague accidentally pours a container of hot liquid over their hand. What first aid measures do you take?

5. What are the contra indications for using vacuum-assisted wound closure?

6. You wish to change practice on a surgical ward and introduce the use of a specific post-operative dressing which is water-proof and vapour permeable. This new dressing is more expensive. What arguments would you put forward to justify the change of dressings?

7. A patient in your care is complaining that her wound is becoming 'smelly' which is making her feel very embarrassed. Which of the following would you consider as the appropriate first steps to take in order to eliminate odour?

   a) Obtain a wound swab ☐
   b) Prescribe antibiotics ☐
   c) Examine the wound for signs of infection ☐
   d) Thoroughly cleanse the wound in order to remove excess
      exudate and wound debris ☐
   e) Re-evaluate frequency of dressing changes ☐
   f) Re-evaluate appropriateness of dressing in use ☐

8. The following cells are all involved in the wound healing process. Match them with their functions:

a) mast cells	a)	phagocytosis
b) histamine	b)	collagen synthesis
c) neutrophils	c)	wound contraction
d) macrophages	d)	releases histamine
e) fibroblasts	e)	generates new epidermis
f) myofibroblasts	f)	triggers vasodilation
g) epithelial cells	g)	first defence leucocytes

9. A patient in your care presents with a heavily exuding venous leg ulcer which is causing maceration to the surrounding skin. Which of the following are probable causes for this high exudate loss?

a) infection ☐
b) hydrostatic pressure ☐
c) pain ☐
d) inappropriate dressings and/or wear time ☐
e) sleeping in a chair ☐
f) diabetes ☐
g) lack of compression ☐

10. You are looking after a patient who presents with a small sacral, cavity pressure ulcer. The wound bed is sloughy and there is a moderate exudate loss. Following assessment, your criteria for appropriate dressing(s) include the following: absorbent, conformable, ability to de-slough the wound. Suggest suitable dressing types that fulfil this criteria.

Answers

1. d) 2. Grade 1
3. Loss of appetite, unintentional weight loss of more than 5% in last one to two months, ability to obtain and prepare food
4. ABC assessment, irrigate with cool water for ten to twenty minutes, carefully remove wet clothing, elevate arm, reassure, arrange specialist assessment of extent of damage
5. Malignancy, untreated osteomylitis, exposed blood vessels and organs, non-enteric and unexplored fisutulas, dry necrotic tissue
6. Reduction in pain and anxiety, reduced need for and cost of analgesia, improved infection prevention, increased patient satisfaction, reduction in skin damage and blistering, improved exudate management, less frequent dressing changes
7. c-f, swabbing wounds and prescribing anti-biotics should not be undertaken routinely
8. f/c, d/a, b/f, a/d, e/b, g/e
9. a), b), d), e), g)
10. Primary: hydrogels, alginates, hydrocolloids, hydrofibre; Secondary: Foams

Glossary of terms

Acute wound

A wound that progresses through the normal stages of healing without hindrance

Ankle brachial pressure index (ABPI

Index of arterial efficiency obtained using Doppler ultrasound. The highest pressure reading from the ankle is divided by the highest pressure measurement from the arm. The normal ABPI is 1.0

Alginate dressing

Highly absorbent dressing derived from seaweed

Allografts

Tissue taken from one individual for use on another

Angiography

Diagnostic test whereby a radio-opaque dye is injected into the arteries proximal to any problem area and images recorded of its passage

Autologous grafts

Harvesting of an individual's own skin

Autolysis

The means by which the body's own defence mechanism produces enzymes which break down and remove necrotic tissue

Bacterial load

Amount of bacteria present in the wound bed

Biosurgery

Use of maggot (larvae) to debride necrotic tissue in wound

Body mass index (BMI)

Height for weight ratio expresses as: weight (present)/height (squared).
- Average range   =   20–25
- Under nutrition =   19 and below
- Over nutrition =   30 an above

Cavity

Hollowed out area of tissue loss. May occur following infection, debridement or pressure damage

Cellulitis

Inflammation and infection of skin, commonly caused by *Streptoccoci* and *Staphyloccocus aureus*. Presenting features include redness, swelling, heat and pain

Charcot's foot	Condition where pedal arch of foot collapses. A condition that is related to diabetes
Chemical debridement	Use of chemicals (varidase, hydrogen peroxide) to remove necrotic and sloughy tissue
Chronic oedema	Swelling of greater than three months duration
Chronic wound	A wound that does not proceed through the normal stages of healing in an orderly fashion but becomes stuck in the process and so does not proceed to full healing
Coagulation	Area of non-viable tissue which is at the centre of a burn injury
Collagen	A protein that is produced by the body and forms the basic building matrix and is therefore necessary for wound repair. It is secreted by fibroblasts during the reconstructive phase of healing
Compression bandages	Bandage systems used to aid venous return and in the management of chronic oedema and lymphoedema. They are available as short-stretch or long-stretch and can be used as part of a multi-layer combination
Contact inhibition	The point when proliferating epithelial cells meet and stop as the wound repair is completed
Coronal plane	Divides the body into front and back
Delayed primary closure	Skin closure following surgery is delayed for a number of days, usually as a result of high risk of infection
Dermo-epidermal junction	Basal membrane between epidermis and dermis. Can be subject to injury from shearing forces
Diabetes mellitus	A disease in which the regulation of glucose within the body is impaired
Diabetic neuropathy	Loss of sensation and vasomotor control as a result of nerve damage from glucose. Both sensory and motor nerves may be effected

Dehiscence

Breakdown and separation of surgical wound edges due to infection. May be either partial or complete

Doppler ultrasound

Hand-held Doppler ultrasound probe used in the assessment of vascular function. Is used in order to obtain the ankle brachial pressure index (ABPI) as a precursor to the application of compression bandages

Entonox

A mixture of nitrous oxide and air. Can be used as a short-term analgesia for procedural pain, eg. changing wound dressings

Epithelial tissue

Tissue that is present in final stages of healing and which forms new epidermis

Erythema

Redness of skin as a result of inflammation and infection or as a response to pressure loading of the skin

Eschar

Dry, hard, necrotic or dead tissue

Exudate

Serous fluid present in wound. The amount of exudate will depend on stage of healing and whether any infection or oedema are present. Exudate is necessary for maintaining a moist wound bed and for healing as it contains growth factors. Excessive exudate will lead to maceration and excoriation

Fibroblasts

Cells that enter the wound in the reconstruction phase. They secrete collagen fibres to produce the basic building matrix

First intention healing

In first intention healing (sometimes referred to as primary healing), wound edges are re-approximated by sutures or clips which accelerate wound healing

Foam dressing

Highly absorbent dressing made of hydrophillic polyurethane or other compounds

Friction forces

Forces that occur when two surfaces rub together. This is enhanced in the presence of heat and moisture

Full-thickness wound

A wound that involves loss of the epidermis, dermis, subcutaneous tissue or even deeper structures such as muscle. Bone may be visible

Fungating tumours	See malignant wound
Granulation tissue	Moist, red tissue composed of capillary loops, supporting collagen and ground substance, produced in the granulation stage of healing to fill any defect
Healing cascade	Sequence of triggered events which take place following tissue injury which causes bleeding
Hydrocolloid dressing	Absorbent, occlusive dressing made from a mixture of pectin, sodium carboxymethyl cellulose and elastomers
Hydrogel dressing	Gel which consists of approximately 70% of water and other compounds. Available in amorphous gel or sheet dressing
Hydrofibre dressing	Highly absorbent dressing, chemically similar to a hydrocolloid
Reactive hyperaemia	Bright red flush of the skin associated with the increased volume of the pulse on the release of an obstruction to the circulation, or a vascular flush following the release of an occlusion of the circulation which is a normal response to incoming arterial blood. This will fade fairly quickly
Blanching hyperaemia	The phenomena whereby skin blanches or whitens if light finger pressure is applied to an area of reactive hyperaemia, indicating that the patient's microcirculation is intact
Non-blanching hyperaemia	Indicated when there is no skin colour change of the erythema when light finger pressure is applied, indicating a degree of microcirculatory disruption. often associated with other clinical signs, such as blistering, induration and oedema
Integumentary system	The body system which comprises the skin and the structures that lie within it
Infected tissue	Tissue that has been invaded by micro-organisms that have elicited a host response. The classic signs of infected tissue include pain, swelling, redness and purulent discharge

Inflammation

Normal response to tissue trauma in which the body's defence forces are alerted and mobilised. The signs of inflammation include redness, heat, pain and swelling. Many of these reactions are initiated by the release of histamine from mast cells

Leg ulceration

An area of discontinuity of epidermis or dermis on the lower leg or feet existing for longer than six weeks

Leptospermum honey

Honey from New Zealand and Australia – often referred to as Manuka honey

Leucocytes

White blood cells of which there are three types. Polymorphonuclear cells, monocytes and lymphocytes (includes eosinophils, neutrophils). Some of these cells are responsible for defence at time of injury

Maceration

Water-logged, over-hydrated skin as a result of prolonged exposure to moisture. May appear white in appearance and is prone to damage and breakdown

Macrophage

Phagocytic cells which are able to ingest debris and bacteria. They are also important chemotatic agents in that they release chemicals that stimulate further stages of wound healing

Malignant wound

Area of malignant growth and ulceration. Infiltration of malignant cells into the skin and supporting structures can result in a fungating tumour

Malodorous wound

A wound with an offensive smell due to either specific or excessive amounts of bacteria in the wound and/or presence of necrotic tissue

Maturation

Final phase of wound healing in which the newly laid down tissue is reorganised and contracts in size to form final scar

Mixed aetiology

A condition that has a number of causes. In leg ulceration this may mean the presence of both venous insufficiency and arterial disease

Moist wound healing

Healing system that utilises moisture to facilitate an increased healing rate

Myofibroblasts	Specialist fibroblasts which have contractile properties. They are able reduce the size of the wound by pulling the edges together
Necrotic tissue	Dead tissue that is either black, brown or grey in colour and may vary in consistency
Neutrophils	(see leucocytes)
Occlusive dressing	A permeable or semi-impermeable dressing that prevents the passage of bacteria
Palmar surface	Palm of the hand
Partial-thickness wound	A wound that involves loss of epidermal and dermal cells
Phagocytosis	The breaking down and removal of debris, other dead cells and bacteria by cells through ingestion
Plantar surface	Sole of the foot
Pressure	Perpendicular load of force exerted on a unit of area
Pressure ulceration	Localised cellular damage to the skin and underlying tissues caused by pressure, friction and shear. Usually occurs on bony prominences such as sacrum, trochanters and heels
Primary wound closure	Wound closure achieved by bringing together skin edges with good apposition following surgery
Proteolytic enzymes	Enzymes that promote the breakdown of proteins and dead tissue during the healing process
Reconstruction	The building of new tissue using a matrix of collagen. This stage takes place when all debris has been removed from the wound
Re-epithelialisation	Phase of wound healing in which epithelial cells are able to migrate across the wound once it has been sufficiently filled with new granulation tissue
Sagittal plane	Divides the body into left and right

Second intention healing	The wound is not closed and healing is achieved by the formation of granulation tissue to fill any defect Epithelial cells are able to migrate over this
Secondary closure	Skin closure following surgery is delayed for a longer period of ten to fourteen days
Sharp debridement	Removal of dead tissue using a scalpel or scissors
Shear forces	Force that results in layers of tissue moving in opposite planes
Sinus	An abnormal blind-ended tract that is present between the skin or wound and the deeper tissues
Slough	Collection of dead cells, and wound debris. It is usually yellow in appearance and may vary in consistency
Stasis	Area of tissue following burn injury that is viable but fragile, and is at high risk due to reduced tissue perfusion
Strike through	Leakage of exudate through to outer layer of a dressing. This is caused by either the inability of the dressing to cope with the level of exudate or because the time between dressing changes is too long
Superficial wound	A wound that only involves loss of epidermal cells
Surgical debridement	Removal of dead tissue by surgery using either general or local anaesthetic
Surgical wound	A wound formed from an incision that has been undertaken in a sterile environment
Tissue engineering	The development of new materials or devices capable of specific interactions with biological tissues
Vapour permeable	A dressing that is able to allow the passage of gases and water vapour through it. Vapour permeable film dressings are transparent dressings with a high vapour permeable transmission rate

Venous insufficiency/disease   The valves in the leg become inadequate leading to pooling of blood in the lower leg

Wound bed preparation   The management of a wound in order to accelerate endogenous healing or to facilitate the effectiveness of other methods of wound healing

Reference

Collins F, Hampton S, White R (2002) *A–Z Dictionary of Wound Care*. Quay Books, MA Healthcare Limited, Dinton, Salisbury

Further sources of information, societies and Government internet addresses

National Pressure Ulcer Advisory Panel (US)	www.npuap.org
European Pressure Ulcer Advisory Panel	www.epuap.com
Wound Care Society (UK)	www/woundcaresociety.org
Tissue Viability Society (UK)	www.tvs.org.uk
Leg Ulcer Forum	www.legulcerforum.org
World Wide Wounds	www.smtl.co.uk/world-wide-wounds
Cochrane collaboration	www.cochrane.org
Scottish Intercollegiate Guidelines Network (SIGN)	www.signs.ac.uk
Society for Vascular Surgery	www.vascsurg.org
Podiatry online	www.footdoc.com/footman.pdonline.html
BMC Complementary and Alternative Medicine	www.biomedcentral.com
Department of Health	www.doh.gov.uk
Commission for Health Improvement	www.chi.gov.uk
Royal College of Nursing	www.rcn.org.uk
National Institute for Clinical Excellence	www.nice.org.uk

Appendix 1: Wound care treatment plan/wound assessment and evaluation record

Elderly Directorate Version

SOUTH BIRMINGHAM PRIMARY CARE NHS TRUST

WOUND CARE TREATMENT PLAN

Name & address / Pnum

Site of Wound

Date of plan	Date of plan	Date of plan
Dressing frequency/ weartime	Dressing frequency/ weartime	Dressing frequency/ weartime
Primary aim (circle) Debride Deslough Promote granulation Promote epithelialisation Control infection Other (state)	Primary aim (circle) Debride Deslough Promote granulation Promote epithelialisation Control infection Other (state)	Primary aim (circle) Debride Deslough Promote granulation Promote epithelialisation Control infection Other (state)
CLEANSING REGIME Product Method	CLEANSING REGIME Product Method	CLEANSING REGIME Product Method
SKIN CARE Product Method	SKIN CARE Product Method	SKIN CARE Product Method
DEBRIDEMENT PROCEDURE Required Yes/No Product Method	DEBRIDEMENT PROCEDURE Required Yes/No Product Method	DEBRIDEMENT PROCEDURE Required Yes/No Product Method

Elderly Directorate Version

BIRMINGHAM SPECIALIST COMMUNITY HEALTH NHS TRUST

WOUND CARE TREATMENT PLAN

PRIMARY WOUND CARE Product Method	PRIMARY WOUND CARE Product Method	PRIMARY WOUND CARE Product Method
SECONDARY DRESSING/ FIXATIVE Product Method	SECONDARY DRESSING/ FIXATIVE Product Method	SECONDARY DRESSING/ FIXATIVE Product Method
PAIN MANAGEMENT Product Frequency Special Instructions	PAIN MANAGEMENT Product Frequency Special Instructions	PAIN MANAGEMENT Product Frequency Special Instructions
COMPRESSION YES/NO Product Special Instructions	COMPRESSION YES/NO Product Special Instructions	COMPRESSION YES/NO Product Special Instructions
OTHER INSTRUCTIONS	OTHER INSTRUCTIONS	OTHER INSTRUCTIONS
ASSESSOR Name Signature	ASSESSOR Name Signature	ASSESSOR Name Signature

Elderly Directorate Version

SOUTH BIRMINGHAM PRIMARY CARE NHS TRUST

WOUND ASSESSMENT AND EVALUATION RECORD

Patient Name & Address / Pnum	Type of Wound
Length of time wound present	If pressure sore circle below
Site of Wound	**Ischial tuberosity** **Heel** **Sacrum** **Other (state)** **Trochanter**

Factors that may delay healing

Medication	Allergies	Anaemia
Diabetes	Immobility	Poor Nutritional status
Client has difficulty with compliance	Others	

DATE							

1. Size (cm)

Length (max)							
Breadth (max)							
Depth (max)							
Grade if pressure sore)							

2. Wound bed; estimate %

Necrotic							
Sloughly							
Granulating							
Epithelialising							

3. Exudate

Colour							
Consistency							
Amount: Minimal							
Moderate							
Heavy							

DATE						

4. Odour

None							
Some							
Offensive							

5. Pain 0 - 10: 0= No Pain 10= Severe Pain

Pre analgesia score							
Post analgesia score							
None							
At dressing change							
Intermittent							
Continuous							

6. Condition of surrounding skin

Macerated							
Oedematous							
Eczema							
Fragile							
Dry/Scaling							
Healthy/Intact							

7. Infection

Clinical signs presents							
Suspected (eg non-healing)							
Wound swab sent							
Organism identified							

Tracing done							

Assessor							

Signature							

Appendix 2: Wound treatment matrix

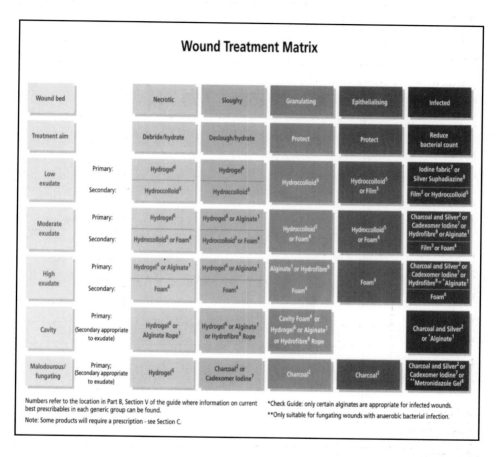

Wound Treatment Matrix

Wound bed		Necrotic	Sloughy	Granulating	Epithelialising	Infected
Treatment aim		Debride/hydrate	Deslough/hydrate	Protect	Protect	Reduce bacterial count
Low exudate	Primary:	Hydrogel[6]	Hydrogel[6]	Hydroccolloid[5]	Hydrocolloid[5] or Film[3]	Iodine fabric[7] or Silver Suphadiazine[8]
	Secondary:	Hydroccolloid[5]	Hydroccolloid[5]			Film[3] or Hydroccolloid[5]
Moderate exudate	Primary:	Hydrogel[6]	Hydrogel[6] or Alginate[1]	Hydroccolloid[5] or Foam[4]	Hydroccolloid[5] or Foam[4]	Charcoal and Silver[2] or Cadexomer Iodine[7] or Hydrofibre[8] or Alginate[1]
	Secondary:	Hydroccolloid[5] or Foam[4]	Hydroccolloid[5] or Foam[4]			Film[3] or Foam[4]
High exudate	Primary:	Hydrogel[6] or Alginate[1]	Hydrogel[6] or Alginate[1]	Alginate[1] or Hydrofibre[8]	Foam[4]	Charcoal and Silver[2] or Cadexomer Iodine[7] or Hydrofibre[8] or *Alginate[1]
	Secondary:	Foam[4]	Foam[4]	Foam[4]		Foam[4]
Cavity	Primary: (Secondary appropriate to exudate)	Hydrogel[6] or Alginate Rope[1]	Hydrogel[6] or Alginate[1] or Hydrofibre[8] Rope	Cavity Foam[4] or Hydrogel[6] or Alginate[1] or Hydrofibre[8] Rope		Charcoal and Silver[2] or *Alginate[1]
Malodourous/ fungating	Primary; (Secondary appropriate to exudate)	Hydrogel[6]	Charcoal[2] or Cadexomer Iodine[7]	Charcoal[2]	Charcoal[2]	Charcoal and Silver[2] or Cadexomer Iodine[7] or **Metronidazole Gel[8]

Numbers refer to the location in Part B, Section V of the guide where information on current best prescribables in each generic group can be found.

Note: Some products will require a prescription - see Section C.

*Check Guide: only certain alginates are appropriate for infected wounds.
**Only suitable for fungating wounds with anaerobic bacterial infection.

Produced by the Birmingham Community Wound Formulary Working Party

Appendix 3: European Pressure Ulcer Advisory Panel Guide to Pressure Ulcer Grading

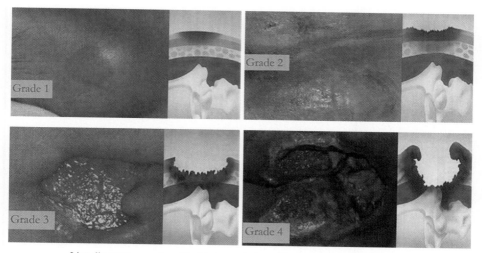

Line diagrams reproduced by kind permission of Huntleigh Healthcare Limited

Appendix 4: Treatment of a wound infection in a patient with mantle cell lymphoma

This case study examines the impact of a severe wound infection on a patient undergoing chemotherapy for the treatment of mantle cell lymphoma. The study illustrates how life threatening an infection can become in a patient whose body is compromised as a consequence of both disease and chemotherapy treatment. A number of specialist products were required in order to overcome the infection, debride and heal the wound. These included larval therapy, vacuum-assisted closure and Leptospermum honey.

Mantle lymphoma is a non-Hodgkin's lymphoma and is sometimes referred to as 'intermediate lymphocytic lymphoma'. Mason and Gatter (1998) state that it has derived its name from its histological appearance of small- to medium-sized cells which have a nodular or mantle zone growth pattern. Mantle cell lymphoma predominantly affects males with a median age of sixty years and it frequently spreads to blood and bone marrow. It is quite aggressive and long-term survival is rare. The disease usually presents with lymphadenopathy, but may be found at extranodal sites, notably the gastrointestinal tract (lymphomatous polyposis).

This case study describes the treatment of a patient with mantle cell lymphoma who acquired a severe wound infection and abdominal cellulitis following a lymph node biopsy from the right thigh. A range of treatment options were used to heal the wound, including larvae therapy (LarvE), vacuum-assisted closure (VAC), and Leptospermum honey. The outcome was very favourable, with complete healing being achieved within fourteen weeks.

Case report

The patient

A sixty-three-year-old man was referred to Salisbury District Hospital for chemotherapy treatment of his mantle cell lymphoma using a combination therapy known as CHOP (*Table Appendix 4.1*).

Three days before the administration of the CHOP therapy, he underwent a biopsy of three large lymph nodes from his right thigh. Following the removal of the sutures from the biopsy site one week later, the incision site appeared inflamed and tender. Within three days this had progressed to a deep cavity with necrotic tissue present and cellulitis which extended across the whole of the abdomen. A wound swab was later to show the presence of methicillin-resistant *Staphylococcus aureus* (MRSA), *Staphylococcus aureus* and *Enterococcus spp.* Blood results showed that the patient was very compromised with haemoglobin 5g/l, white blood cells of 0.6 109/l, neutrophils of 0.5 109/l, platelets of 3.0 109/l, a C-reactive protein of 354mg/l and an albumin level of 25g/l.

Wound management

The initial management consisted of the administration of platelets to boost his depleted level and to commence on gentamicin in an attempt to eradicate the infection. He was then taken to theatre for exploration and cleaning of the groin wound, which was approximately 12cm in length and extended down to the peritoneum. The wound was packed with an alginate (Kaltostat, manufactured by ConvaTec) intraoperatively which was later changed to gauze soaked with betadine. It was at this stage that the tissue viability service became involved and a thorough reassessment of the patient undertaken, involving wound management and nutrition.

Table Appendix 4.1: CHOP chemotherapy	
Indications	
High grade/intermediate non-Hodgkin's lymphoma. Given three-weekly for six cycles	
Drug combination	
Cyclophosphamide	$750mg/m^2$ IV bolus — day 1
Doxorubicin	$50mg/m^2$ IV bolus — day 1
Vincristine	$1.4mg/m^2$ IV bolus — day 1
Prednisolone	100mg orally — day 1–5
Side-effects	
Can cause nausea	
Myelosuppression	
Alopecia	
Steroid side-effects: retarded wound healing, reduced tensile strength and inhibition of collagen synthesis (Miller, 1999)	
Cardiac toxicity with accumulated doses of doxorubicin	
Peripheral neuropathy from the vincristine	
IV = intravenous	

Larvae therapy

Despite surgical debridement the wound still remained necrotic (*Figure Appendix 4.1*) so larvae therapy was commenced. The platelet level had risen by that stage to 181mg/l but the wound was still carefully monitored for bleeding.

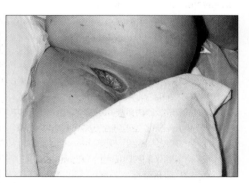

Two applications were applied, but the wound was so wet that they had limited success. A foam cavity dressing was placed in the cavity on the second application with the aim of absorbing some of the excess exudate. Unfortunately, this was unsuccessful as the maggots migrated into the dressing. As the amount of exudate and lymph from the cellulitis was becoming excessive and problematic another approach was required.

Figure Appendix 4.1: Wound before larval therapy, showing extent of tissue breakdown, necrosis and surrounding cellulitis

Vacuum-assisted closure (VAC)

The second approach was to use VAC. The perceived advantages of this is its ability to draw off the excessive amounts of exudate (and thus reduce the oedema), open up the blood supply to the wound and also provide a closed system to reduce the risk of further infection. At this stage, the wound still contained slough and necrotic tissue and had a heavy exudate level (*Figure Appendix 4.2*).

The amount of consistency of the exudate again presented initial problems. The canister full alarm on the machine was being set off constantly and, on close inspection, it was found that the lymph from the wound was being drawn off in an aerosol effect. This was spraying directly into the canister sensor and setting it off. To overcome this technical problem the pressure was reduced to 75mmHg and the tubing elevated above the machine to encourage downward drainage and not directly into the sensor head.

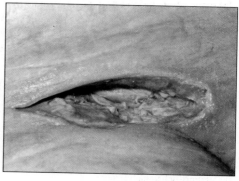

Figure Appendix 4.2: Wound before vacuum-assisted closure

Significant improvements both within the wound and to the surrounding cellulitis were noted within one week. The exudate had reduced in amount and was more viscous as it contained less lymph fluid. The VAC settings were increased and no further problems were experienced with the machine.

The patient was discharged home after two weeks but attended as a day patient for the administration of his chemotherapy. The community nursing staff undertook the dressing procedures and the clinical nurse specialist assisted while he was in hospital. It was explained that the rate of healing might be negatively affected once chemotherapy started.

Although the rate did slow down slightly, it never became static as first envisaged. After seven weeks of VAC therapy the wound was found to be too small for the VAC dressing to be comfortable for the patient. He also wanted to return to work part-time and did not want the inconvenience of a machine.

The wound was very clean but still concave (*Figure Appendix 4.3*) and it remained at continued risk of infection as a result of the chemotherapy. At this stage, the patient's haemoglobin was 117g/l, platelets were 117g/l and his neutrophils were 2.4g/l, which left him still compromised. It was decided to use an antibacterial product that would still stimulate healing. Following success with another infected wound a honey dressing was chosen.

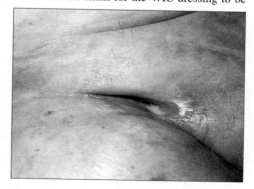

Figure Appendix 4.3: Significant wound closure following seven weeks of vacuum-assisted wound closure

Leptospermum honey

Leptospermum honey was applied to the wound on a daily basis. It is supplied in 50g tubes, which are gamma irradiated (Medihoney, Australia). Currently, this honey does not have a product license for use in wound management in the UK.

Approximately 15–20g of the honey was applied to the wound, which was then covered with a simple non-adherent dressing pad (Telfa). This was a simple, daily procedure, which was undertaken by the community nursing team. Once the wound had decreased significantly in size, the patient undertook this procedure himself and then later his wife was able to do it. A good rate of healing continued, with no adverse events and the wound was completely healed and free of MRSA, *Staphylococcus aureus* and *Enterococcus spp.* within four weeks of starting the honey treatment (*Figure Appendix 4.4*).

A total of six courses of CHOP chemotherapy had been given during the wound healing period, which would have been expected to have had an adverse effect on wound healing, but fortunately this was not the case. Despite the severity of the wound and the administration of a further five courses of CHOP chemotherapy, the wound healed completely within fourteen weeks, which is a relatively short period.

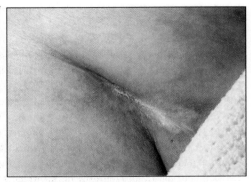

Figure Appendix 4.4: Wound after fourteen weeks. Total closure is achieved following use of Leptospermum honey

Discussion

The chemotherapy, together with the patient's disease state, resulted in the patient's severe wound infection. The immune disruption caused by the disease will have increased his susceptibility to infection while the combination chemotherapy will have lowered this resistance even further.

As can be seen in *Table Appendix 4.1*, each of the drugs has significant side-effects and is toxic to bone marrow. Prednisolone, although not classed as an anti-cancer agent, has been shown to improve significantly both the response and survival rate when used in addition to vincristine and procarbazine in the treatment of lymphoma (Calvert and McElwain, 1988). The low albumin level of 25g/l indicated a degree of malnutrition and would also have presented as a major impairment to wound healing.

When bone marrow toxicity occurs, it results in a fall of the white cell and platelet counts of the patient at varying times (seven to twenty-eight days) after treatment, and anaemia may also occur (Calvert and McElwain, 1988). This is clearly demonstrated by the patient's blood picture at the presentation of the infection. Not only would the patient's clinical picture have resulted in the infection because of the presence of white cells, but also it would have impeded subsequent healing for a variety of reasons.

During the initial stages of wound healing there is a rapid proliferation of a host of cell types. These cells have a high mitotic and proliferation rate and are also affected by the chemotherapy. As Mulder *et al* (1998) have described, suppression of the haemopietic tissues could also disrupt wound healing either by a lack of initiation of subsequent cascades as a result of decreased platelet degranulation, or through an increased risk of infection secondary to leucopenia. Corticosteroids also have a major effect on wound healing as they inhibit fibroblast function and subsequent collagen synthesis.

It is felt that the treatment choices influence the outcome greatly. Each treatment has been shown to be effective against infection, necrosis and to stimulate healing.

Clinical experience has shown that larval therapy is effective in removing necrotic tissue and combating infection as a result of the secretion of a powerful mixture of proteolytic enzymes. The main use of larval therapy is in the treatment of necrotic or sloughy wounds such as pressure and leg ulcers. Jones *et al* (1998) have described their use in osteomyelitis, malignant wounds,